PRAISE FOR
DIABETES AND ME

"All parents of children with diabetes should read this book! As a former pediatric nurse and the mother of a son who has type 1 diabetes, I have seen firsthand how devastating a child's diabetes diagnosis can be for families—and I know how helpful it is to hear from others who are on the same journey. Wendy's story is captivating, and she includes practical advice alongside compelling anecdotes about the challenges of navigating the ups and downs of diabetes. She also explains the medical aspects of the disease in a way that's clear and easy to understand."

—**Madeline Bell**, President and CEO, Children's Hospital of Philadelphia

"'Your child has diabetes.' Hearing those words can strike fear into the heart of any parent. Type 1 diabetes is not just a challenge for an individual, it affects entire families. In addition to the uncertainty that a diagnosis can bring, learning how to manage blood sugar with insulin is a lifelong burden. Wendy's lifelong journey shows just how important family is—starting with her father's own experience with type 1 diabetes and continuing with the unwavering support of her husband and daughter. This family support has been critical to helping her through the emotional, psychological, and physical ups and downs of the disease over a lifetime.

The past one hundred years has taken us from the discovery of insulin, a treatment given by syringes sterilized at home in boiling water, to the advent of insulin pumps and automatic blood sugar monitors. Wendy has seen it all in her lifetime. Her dedication to type 1 diabetes education and working to create a better world for patients is unparalleled—as is her spirit.

Hearing those words no longer is about fear . . . it's about hope for a bright future. This book shows just how possible it is to persevere and live a long, fulfilling life with type 1 diabetes."

—**Kupper A. Wintergerst, MD,** Wendy L. Novak Chair of Pediatric Diabetes Care and Clinical Research and pediatric endocrinologist with Norton Children's Endocrinology, affiliated with the UofL School of Medicine

"Wendy Novak is a testimony to accepting the cards one is dealt and surpassing all expectations and odds. She is the embodiment of resilience, kindness, acceptance, and the human spirit. This book is a must-read for the millions of people who live with diabetes but also for everyone who has personal challenges they must face. She is by their side every step of the way when recounting her own very personal story."

—**Elaine and Ken Langone**

DIABETES AND ME

DIABETES AND ME

Living a Healthy and Empowered Life in the Face of Diabetes

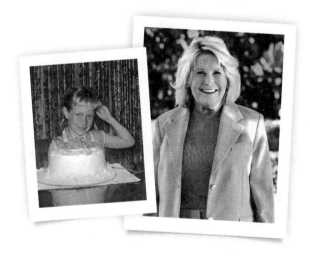

WENDY LOUISE NOVAK

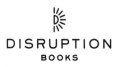

DISRUPTION
BOOKS

Austin   New York

Published by Disruption Books
New York, New York
www.disruptionbooks.com

Distributed by Disruption Books

For information about special discounts for bulk purchases, please contact
Disruption Books at info@disruptionbooks.com.

Cover design by Liz Driesbach
Book design by Brian Phillips Design

Library of Congress Cataloging-in-Publication Data is available

Printed in the United States of America

Print ISBN: 978-1-63331-080-3
eBook ISBN: 978-1-63331-081-0

First Edition

Dedicated to my loving husband, David,
and cherished daughter, Ashley, who are
always by my side when I need them the most.
I love them with all my heart.

CONTENTS

Foreword by David Novak   xi

Chapter 1: **Awareness**   1

Chapter 2: **Identity**   15

Chapter 3: **Independence**   31

Chapter 4: **Risk and Reward**   47

Chapter 5: **Adjustment**   63

Chapter 6: **Acceptance**   77

Chapter 7: **Perseverance**   93

Chapter 8: **Renewal**   105

Afterword: Giving Back   115

Acknowledgments   121

About the Institute   125

About the Author   127

FOREWORD

WHEN I MET MY WIFE, WENDY, in the early 1970s, she never would have considered writing a book about having type 1 diabetes. In fact, it was probably the last thing she would ever do. That was information she liked to keep private. Our first real fight, not long after we were married, happened because I casually mentioned her condition to someone at a cocktail party. She was not happy about that. She was right that I shouldn't have said anything. It was her business to tell, not mine. The thing is, she really never told it, not to many people and not for many years anyway.

But she's telling it now, and she's doing it for a reason that's quintessentially Wendy: to help other people. And there are a lot of people out there who could use some help in this area. Nearly two million people in the United States are living with type 1 diabetes, according to the American Diabetes Association. Tens xii • DIABETES AND ME

of millions more have type 2 diabetes. In total, individuals with diabetes make up more than 11 percent of the US population.

The fact that Wendy has always been so other-directed is only part of the reason why she almost never talked about her diabetes. The bigger reason was because that's how she grew up. She inherited the condition from her father, who was diagnosed at a time when insulin treatment was still quite new. Back then, many considered diabetes a death sentence or, at the very least, something that made people fragile and sickly. Her dad didn't want anyone to know because he didn't want people to think of him that way. As it turned out, he lived many years with diabetes—and he had an active and successful life too—but if his employers had ever found out about his condition, they could have stifled his career or even fired him. Being open about having diabetes at that time in history could have, quite literally, kept him from providing for his family.

But times have changed since then. Not only have attitudes changed, but the medications and technologies to treat diabetes have evolved considerably. It's now far from a dire diagnosis. It's something that, with the right kind of care and attention, doesn't need to hold people back from living their lives fully, joyfully, and with real purpose.

Wendy has decided it's time to tell the story that her dad would never tell. She no longer wants to keep her condition a secret. Instead, she wants to show people what life is really like for people living with diabetes and to prove that, while it has more than its share of challenges, it can be pretty darn amazing, just like it has been for her.

Wendy has a real story to tell too. By most standards, we've lived a pretty storied life. Beyond that, I've had the good fortune of meeting a lot of highly accomplished people over the years, but I've never known anyone to display the level of resilience, inner strength, and grace under the toughest of circumstances that my wife Wendy has shown over and over and over again.

I've learned from Wendy that when you have something like diabetes, you never get a day off. I was diagnosed with cancer several years ago, but as difficult as that was, I was conscious of the fact that it's something you can recover from. Diabetes isn't. It's ever present. Because of it, she has been knocked down in her life so many times that both of us have lost count. I've come far too close to losing her more than once. Even as she was in the midst of writing this book, she suffered a stroke and afterward took a bad fall and broke her shoulder. The injury was so painful, she could barely move for weeks, and the pain medications she was given left her with hallucinations, a likely complication of her condition since medications can affect people with diabetes differently. Still, she fought back. She recovered from her injury, regained her mobility, and went on to finish this book, all while managing her condition. She is, quite simply, a warrior and an inspiration to many people. She certainly is to me.

Someone asked her not long ago if her father would have been proud of her for writing this book. She said yes and then no. He would have been proud of her for showing the world that she can do anything that anyone else can do, that her diabetes, while it needs to be managed, is not a limitation. On the other hand, xiv • DIABETES AND ME

she wasn't so certain that he'd be proud of her for revealing the family secret.

But she's doing it anyway because that's Wendy: caring, capable, strong, and fiercely independent. When she puts her mind to something, there's no stopping her. I've had the good fortune of sharing this journey with her for nearly fifty years, and I'm thrilled that she's now sharing some of it with you. I hope it will paint a picture of the realities, challenges, and possibilities of having diabetes, and if you're one of the thirty-seven-plus million people in the United States living with diabetes, I hope you find in it inspiration to live your life to the fullest. Having diabetes never stopped Wendy, and it can be the same for you.

DAVID NOVAK, founder of David Novak Leadership and cofounder, retired chairman, and CEO of Yum! Brands

Chapter 1

AWARENESS

I **INHERITED A LOT OF THINGS** from my dad, but one of the most notable things is probably my diabetes. As a child he discovered that he had type 1 diabetes, and so did I.

It's funny how the condition can just show up whenever. My dad found out he had it when he was five years old. My brother Jeff, on the other hand, also has the condition, but he wasn't diagnosed until the age of sixty-six. My younger sister Cindy, who does not have diabetes, nonetheless has two children who do, one who was diagnosed at the age of three and the other at the age of twenty-one. The condition was once called juvenile diabetes because it was most commonly diagnosed in children, but as my family can attest, it doesn't always happen that way. In fact, today 50 percent or more of all individuals newly diagnosed with type 1 diabetes are adults. Because the condition can develop at any age, the term "juvenile diabetes" has fallen out of favor, and now it is most commonly referred to as type 1.

I was diagnosed with type 1 diabetes at the age of seven. As my mom remembers it, the family was in the living room watching TV, just like we did most evenings back then, when she suddenly noticed that I kept getting up to use the bathroom. That caught her attention first, and then the next time I was in the bathroom, she could hear me whimpering through the door. I wasn't the type of kid to complain, so that plus the frequent urination, a classic symptom, clued her in.

Of course, she lived with a husband who had diabetes, so she knew the signs. And she had on hand everything she needed to test her suspicion. Back then—this was the late 1950s—people with diabetes would test their blood sugar levels by peeing on yellow test tape. If the test paper turned green, then your blood sugar was high. If it stayed the same color, then it wasn't. The greener it turned, the more sugar you had on board. The next time I had to go to the bathroom, Mom had me use one of Dad's test papers. It turned bright green.

She got me an appointment at the doctor soon after that. He took more accurate measurements, and Mom remembers him saying that my blood sugar wasn't really all that high for a newly diagnosed patient. She had caught it early, a lot earlier than most people who don't know the symptoms to look for, which was fortunate. But that's not what I remember most about that time. What I remember most is having to go to the hospital right away.

I spent several days in the hospital after that. They put me on insulin and taught me how to give myself shots. A nurse had me practice on an orange. I was nervous at first, but it never occurred to me, even at that young age, that I wouldn't be able to do it. My parents acted like it was no big deal, so I guess I believed that too.

Initially, however, I didn't understand that the shots were going to be part of my day-to-day for the rest of my life. Or maybe I just wasn't thinking about it until one day, after I got out of the hospital, I had something of a meltdown. I had been sick before, but it had always been temporary, the kind of thing where you did what was necessary to get through it and get better. This was different, and I got so upset about the fact that I had to keep having these shots day after day after day. I was crying when I said to my parents, "It's not fair."

"You're going to learn pretty quickly that life isn't fair," my dad said to me matter-of-factly in response. "It's not fair, but you're going to have to learn to live your life anyway."

I was still upset, but there was something about the sentiment that made sense to me. It helped me to accept the things I couldn't change (like the fact that I had diabetes and always would) and focus instead on what I could control. That practical perspective has stayed with me. It has often helped me through hard times—often, but not always.

I WAS BORN IN WICHITA, KANSAS, in May of 1952, during the last year of Harry S. Truman's presidency, when *I Love Lucy* was becoming the most-watched show on television, and soon after Mr. Potato Head was introduced to the general public for the very first time. I was the first-born child of Jack and Ann Henderson, who were both from the state of Illinois, though they grew up in separate towns. Mom and Dad met while attending Lake Forest College, a little Presbyterian college located along Lake Michigan, north of Chicago. It's where my mom's parents, her grandparents, and many of her family members had gone. It was something of a family tradition to go to Lake Forest (and one that I would break eighteen years later when I went off to college myself).

My parents got married right after graduation. Mom was only twenty years old at the time, and she had me just two years later, at the age of twenty-two. Four more kids followed in quick succession. All of us except for my youngest sister were born in Wichita, where we lived until I was ten. After me came Cindy two years later, then Jeff two years after that, then Rick less than a year after Jeff, and finally Gretchen, the baby of the family, who was born in Columbia, Missouri.

I imagine that it had to be pretty overwhelming for my mom to have so many kids at such a young age. On top of that, she had both a husband and a daughter with diabetes. And she was living in a time when a lot of the modern conveniences that make parenting just a little easier weren't available. She washed all our diapers by hand, for example, because there weren't disposable ones back then. She made all our meals from scratch and kept the house while Dad worked. She didn't even have a car of her own when I was young. We had just one car that my dad would mostly take for work, so she would have to get a ride with the neighbor across the street to go grocery shopping for the week. But if she was overwhelmed, she never let on. Mom came from Swedish heritage. Her maiden name is Bjorklund, which means "birch tree." True to her name, she was strong, stable, and reliable, just like the hardwood birch.

She was beautiful too. She wore her light-colored hair long and wavy like the Swedish-born actress and singer Ann-Margret, who was known for her roles in films like *Bye Bye Birdie*. If you had seen my mother then, it would come as no surprise that she modeled for Marshall Field's department store when she was in high school.

Dad, by contrast, had dark hair and eyes. He was a good-looking guy of Scottish stock, and I could see why Mom fell in love with him. He was also fiercely independent. I don't remember him ever complaining about his diabetes. Not even once.

Some of that stemmed from the fact that he grew up feeling like there was a stigma attached to having diabetes. He was probably right about that too. He was born in 1927 and developed diabetes five years later. Insulin treatment wasn't even invented until the 1920s, so it hadn't been around long when he started using it. In fact, he had a cousin who had died from diabetes, a fact that had to be on people's minds when he was diagnosed. It may sound funny to say it, but Dad was lucky in a way. If he had developed diabetes a few years earlier, before insulin was available, and if there hadn't been a doctor nearby in Chicago who knew how to treat him, things could have—almost surely would have—turned out very differently.

I'm not sure he always felt so lucky, however. His childhood friends made a big to-do about his condition when he was young. He was from a small community where everyone knew each other and knew each other's business. Some of the kids found out about his diagnosis and would sneak him candy, not understanding that that was probably the worst thing they could do for a kid with diabetes. They did it because they didn't think he would live long, and they felt sorry for him. When my mom found out about Dad's diabetes—which wasn't until after they had been dating for a full year because he intentionally kept it from her just like he did with everybody—her parents were supportive, but some of her friends from college said that she should break things off with him. They were afraid she would have a horrible life if she didn't. It's understandable that people would have believed that then. Until insulin treatment was developed, being diagnosed with the condition meant the person would lead a difficult life and then die young. Of course, insulin treatment changed everything, and Dad's diabetes was well managed at the time, but not everyone understood that. Dad really didn't like having people feel sorry for him, and he never wanted to be treated differently.

Probably because of his experience growing up and because it could be hard, if not impossible, for a person who was known to have diabetes to get a job back then, Dad decided as an adult that he didn't want people to know about his condition. Of course, all us kids knew. After all, we had seen his equipment for managing his condition, and his insulin was kept in the refrigerator right next to what we ate and drank every day. But we only knew the fact of it. We didn't really talk about it, and he never gave himself shots in front of us. And outside the household, it was a well-kept secret.

That was true even after I was diagnosed. We didn't talk about this thing that we both had—and that only we had. None of my siblings ever developed diabetes as children. But we did do one thing together that had to do with our diabetes: In the evenings, Dad and I would boil our needles. We each had our own set of equipment—glass syringes, alcohol swabs, and steel needles—that had to be reused. Of course, before you reused them, you had to sterilize them, so we would stand at the stove together sterilizing our needles in a pot of boiling water, getting them ready for our next round of shots.

One time, when I was around nine years old, my mom woke me up because Dad was having a reaction to his insulin. Sometimes you can accidentally take too much, causing your blood sugar to drop too low, which can make a person feel tired, shaky, and confused. You can even pass out if it gets really low, which is what had happened to my dad. He was unconscious when Mom came to get me, and she wanted me to give him a glucagon shot, which is what you give someone to bring their blood sugar back up in an emergency. I remember feeling groggy, but finally I was able to stick the needle in. Then I stayed with him for a few minutes and talked him out of it. He came to, and I remember him not being very happy, first to have found himself in that position —he liked to think of himself as stable and his condition as well controlled—and second because I had been the one to bring him around. I don't think my fiercely independent father liked the idea that he had needed help from his little girl, whom he wanted to keep all this from to begin with.

The Miracle of Insulin Treatment

The first injection of insulin was given to a fourteen-year-old boy named Leonard Thompson in 1922. He was treated at Toronto General Hospital in Toronto, Canada, and after some trial and error, doctors found a version that worked. Thompson continued to have insulin injections for the rest of his life, which turned out to be a relatively normal one until his death from pneumonia in 1935. Before 1922 there was little in the way of effective treatment for type 1 diabetes. In fact, the only treatment was a starvation diet, which required a person to reduce their carbohydrate and calorie intake to practically nothing. As a result, a diabetes diagnosis was considered an eventual death sentence.

TYPE 1 DIABETES, which is the kind that I have (as opposed to the far more common type 2), is an autoimmune disease where the body's own immune system mistakenly attacks and destroys the insulin-producing cells in a person's pancreas. As a result, the body is unable to produce enough insulin to regulate glucose (sugar) levels in the blood. It's unclear what causes the immune system to malfunction in this way, but there is a genetic component (hence my family tree). The only effective treatment for type 1 diabetes is regular doses of insulin to make up for what the body cannot produce on its own combined with careful monitoring of diet and exercise. If you don't do this, there can be both short- and long-term complications.

I suppose that much of this was explained to me when I was a child, but I don't really remember learning about the details. What I remember most from that time are the shots.

By the time I was diagnosed, a type of long-lasting insulin had been developed, which meant I only had to have shots twice a day on a set schedule, one before breakfast and another before dinnertime. (That was much different than how things were when my dad was young. My mom remembers him having to test his blood sugar regularly throughout the day and then have at least three shots, depending on the results.) I remember we paid $25 for a vial of insulin. That may not sound like a lot now, especially considering the skyrocketing price of insulin these days, which some estimates put as high as $600 per vial, cartridge, or pen, amounting to more than $1,000 a month without insurance unless a person rations their vials. But it felt like a lot of money even then. Thankfully, Dad had a good job working for Sears, Roebuck and Co., so I never had to worry about not having enough.

The insulin came in vials that were kept in the refrigerator. Mine would be in the fridge right next to Dad's. They were basically the same except that I had a lower dosage. Back then insulin came from animals, specifically from the pancreases of pigs and cows. Dad and I both took a version that was a combination of both. One was faster acting, and one was slower acting, so together they made for a long-lasting medication.

I remember those details all these years later probably because from a very young age, I was put in charge of giving myself my own shots. The way I remember it, I did so reliably and without a lot of fuss. And I think my mom would even agree. She always said that I was a "perfect child." I slept through the night as a baby. She was able to toilet train me early. When my younger siblings came along, I would help her look after them even at a very young age. One of my earliest memories, in fact, is of being outside in our front yard with my younger sister Cindy. It was just the two of us, and I remember her crawling toward the street. I ended up sitting on top of her to keep her from getting very far while I yelled for Mom to come outside to help. I don't think I was even school age at the time. It was always my natural instinct to look out for people, and with five kids, Mom could always use the help.

It's hard to know what parts of myself developed just because that's who I am and what parts are because I grew up with diabetes. I know people who identify themselves as chocoholics or having a sweet tooth, for example, but that was never going to be me. Maybe I would have developed a taste for such things if I didn't have diabetes, but I never got the opportunity, so I'll never know. Growing up, I wasn't allowed candy or much in the way of sweets like cake or ice cream. Mom didn't even keep such things in the house, so I never thought about it much except maybe when she'd give me Fig Newtons. They were the only sweets I was allowed, probably because they're really not all that sweet. I was allowed five of them, but I would only eat one or two because I hated them. They just didn't taste like much of a treat. To this day I still hate Fig Newtons.

Instead of having a sweet tooth, I'm a big salad eater. My dad was like that too. His favorite meal was a chef's salad. Do I really like salad, or have I learned to like it because it's good for my blood sugar? There's really no way to tell. Am I a natural care-taker, or did I become one because I had to learn early about the fragility of human life and how to be careful with it? Would I be as resilient a person if I hadn't grown up with this part of me that I had to figure out, work with, or work around to move forward with my life? Would I know how to pick myself up over and over again and move on with things? Would I be as capable? As flexi-ble? Would I have developed the same sense of humor?

Maybe it doesn't really matter. We're all a mix of our genes and our experiences anyway, and diabetes has simply been part of my experience for practically as long as I can remember. Cre-ating a life for myself around my diabetes—or sometimes even in spite of it—is something I've always had to do. But I would never call my diabetes a limitation. My dad taught me that. He always told me that I could do anything I wanted to, that I was capable of anything my friends were capable of, as long as I followed the rules of having diabetes. That was how he put it—I just had to "follow the rules" of diabetes.

As I grew older, however, I wondered how much of that he believed for himself, whether or not he felt like the world was wide open to him as someone who lived with diabetes. He was often a rule follower but not always. He was good about monitor-ing his diet and would eat dinner right at 6 p.m., just like clock-work. He was physically strong and always active, playing tennis and running regularly. All that was good for regulating his blood sugar, but at the same time, he often drank too much, which is not a great habit to have with his condition. And yet, as soon as he got home from work each night, he would fix himself an Early Times bourbon, his favorite value-brand liquor, with just a splash of water. It was his regular habit.

Years later, after my dad passed away, my mother told me that when I got diabetes, he stopped believing in God. He was that heartbroken. He never talked to me about it. He didn't even talk to her about it at the time. It wasn't until many years later that he told her how upset he'd been. And yet, even though he rarely talked about diabetes at all, the one message he instilled in me was that I could do whatever I wanted in life if I just followed the rules. Perhaps he didn't believe it for himself, but he must have believed it for me because the message was hammered home. And looking back on my life now, I think that, most of the time at least, I believed him. I still do.

Type 1 vs. Type 2 Diabetes

TYPE 1	TYPE 2
Once known as "juvenile diabetes"	Once known as "adult-onset diabetes"
Happens when the body's immune system attacks the insulin-producing cells of the pancreas, making it unable to produce enough insulin	Happens when the body becomes resistant to the insulin it produces or when cells respond abnormally to the insulin that is produced
Managed by taking insulin to control blood sugar levels	Managed through medications, lifestyle modifications (diet and exercise), and/or insulin treatment
Affects fewer than 10 percent of people with diabetes	Affects the vast majority of people with diabetes, about 90 percent

Chapter 2

IDENTITY

WHEN I THINK ABOUT my childhood, I think of myself as a frequently sick kid. Some of my earliest memories are of being in the hospital. I had pneumonia five times by the time I was five years old. I also had asthma, and my first trip to the hospital was actually related to that and not to diabetes. I have one of those hazy, early memories of being in an oxygen tent. I have another of a nurse waking me up to give me a shot. To my young eyes, the needle looked enormous, and it frightened me. I must have been very young because I remember being in a crib with the bright hospital lights shining through the slats. Back then parents had to leave their children in the hospital overnight—they couldn't stay with them like they often do today—so I was all alone.

In our house in Wichita, my family had a room upstairs that was the designated sick room. It wasn't just for me either. Whenever one of us kids was ill, we would sleep in the sick room. With four brothers and sisters, someone always seemed to be coming home with some bug or another, and I seemed to catch everything I was exposed to.

I still have a clear image in my mind of that sick room. Mom had put posters on the ceiling of all these popular tourist sites around the world so whoever was in the sick bed had something to look at. She remembers getting them from a travel agency that was swapping out their old posters for new ones and planned to throw away the old ones. The posters were of places like London, Scotland, and the Eiffel Tower in Paris. I would lie there in bed sometimes and pretend I was on a trip. Later in life, it became a real passion of mine to travel, and I like to think it all started there in that sick room.

Mom had her hands full at the time, so I was often alone in that room. The point was to keep me away from the other kids so they didn't get sick too, so I didn't see them often. Still, I didn't think of it as some big, bad place. Being sick didn't particularly bother me. Since I dealt with health issues from such a young age, it always felt like just a fact of life. Once in a while I would have to miss something important, like trick-or-treating for Halloween (I was often sick in the fall for some reason), and that would upset me a little. In fact, in an effort to cheer me up, once a neighbor came to visit me dressed as a clown. I can't remember if it worked. Mostly, though, mine was an attitude of acceptance. I don't remember ever feeling sorry for myself. If I wasn't resting or imagining where I might travel to one day, I would spend my time in the sick room reading. I read a lot in that room. I particularly liked mysteries like the Nancy Drew and the Hardy Boys series.

They kept me occupied through what would sometimes be a full week or even two up in that room.

AT SCHOOL I DIDN'T ALWAYS feel quite as comfortable. When I was in the fifth grade, Dad's job with Sears and Roebuck took us from Wichita to Columbia, Missouri. That meant a new school and new friends. Of course, Mom always let my teachers know about my diabetes in case anything went wrong while I was at school, but I always assumed that none of my classmates knew, and it was never something I thought to talk about, even with the ones I was closest to. I didn't really want them to know, and there was no reason why they had to, so I kept it to myself.

Things changed when I was in the fifth grade. When kids with diabetes start having big hormonal swings as they undergo puberty, it can be more difficult to maintain a stable blood sugar. That's likely what was happening to me when, one day, I got in line to go to the cafeteria for lunch. That's the last thing I remember. Everything after that is a blank up until the moment when the principal came into the cafeteria, scooped me up, and dragged me out kicking and screaming. Apparently, I had been going around the room stealing food off other kids' trays and eating it. They must have thought it was some kind of joke, but I wasn't doing it consciously. My blood sugar had dropped, which can cause real problems when it gets too low and can result in things like confusion, odd behavior, slurred speech, and a loss of coordination among other symptoms. To an outsider, it can even look as if the person is drunk, which of course I wasn't. I was only about ten years old.

Symptoms of Low Blood Sugar

Low blood sugar, also called hypoglycemia, can result from taking too much insulin, not eating enough, consuming too much alcohol, or other factors. It can cause a range of symptoms that result from the brain and body not getting enough glucose (its main source of fuel) to function properly. It's a good idea for family members and friends to be aware of the signs in case a person isn't able to treat the condition themselves. Those symptoms can include the following:

- Hunger
- Dizziness
- Irritability
- Confusion
- Sweating
- Shaking
- Fast heartbeat
- Nervousness or anxiety

When the condition is severe, symptoms can also include the following:

- Weakness
- Difficulty walking
- Difficulty seeing clearly
- Unusual behavior
- Loss of consciousness
- Seizures

Mom came to the school and got me after that. I didn't know what the other kids thought, but I knew a lot of them must have seen what had happened. I was so embarrassed. I didn't want to go back to school the next day. I begged my mother not to make me, but of course she did. I couldn't just hide at home forever, and my return wasn't nearly as bad as I thought it would be. In fact, I don't think anyone even mentioned the incident, not to me anyway, so I went on about my business as if nothing had ever happened.

Looking back now, I realize that my classmates must have known that something was going on. Perhaps a teacher or administrator explained to them why I had behaved so strangely, but if that happened, I didn't hear about it. Maybe I didn't want to know so I could remain blissfully unaware and continue to assume that none of the kids saw me any differently. If that's what it was, then that blissful ignorance disappeared a couple years later when I was in the eighth grade.

At that age, to keep my blood sugar stable, I couldn't wait until lunchtime to eat like the rest of my classmates, so every morning at 10:30 a.m., I would leave class and go down to the cafeteria for a snack. I always tried to be as inconspicuous as possible as I snuck out of the classroom, but some of the kids must have noticed. One day, after I had gone to get my graham cracker or whatever the cafeteria ladies gave me that day, I returned to class, and as soon I walked in the door, I could feel it: everybody was looking at me. It was the first time I ever really felt different from everybody else.

I wasn't there, so I don't know what happened exactly while I was getting my snack. Probably someone asked about me or complained about the special treatment I was getting, and the teacher had to explain why I got to leave class every day when they didn't.

Somehow, though, I knew that my secret was out. Later, that feeling was confirmed when a classmate named Bobby, who I'm pretty sure had a crush on me at the time, came up to me and said, "I'm so sorry for you." I didn't say anything, but I remember thinking, *Why? Why feel sorry for me? Why would you say something like that?* I guess I was like my dad that way: I really didn't like pity.

OF COURSE, NOT ALL MY CHILDHOOD revolved around my health. I was a lot more than just a person with diabetes. I was a lot of things, really, like a big sister. From an early age, I was put in charge of my younger brothers and sisters. My mom always said she did that because I was so responsible for my age, but I think she also desperately needed the help. When we were living in Columbia, Mom would drop us all off at a place called Stephens Lake during the summer. It was a man-made lake with a beach and a swimming area surrounded by a park. At the time, the land was owned by Stephens College, which was a private women's college right in town. I was put in charge of the three little ones, who ranged in age from five to seven years old (my youngest sister, Gretchen, hadn't been born yet), while Mom went back home to do some work around the house or ran errands. I would make sure the kids ate their lunches, usually peanut butter and jelly sandwiches, and that they behaved. I was nine years old.

It was a lot to handle. One time a woman who was there with her own kids came up and said to me, "Wendy, do you realize your brothers are in the lake?" The two youngest ones were in the water all by themselves. I don't know what I'd been doing, but

I hadn't noticed them go in, and I nearly panicked. I got them out quickly enough, and everything was OK, but after that I was always terrified that they were going to drown in that lake.

That was how we spent most of our summer days when we lived in Columbia. We would stay at the lake for the whole day until Mom picked us up around 4 p.m. It wasn't like she was being irresponsible. There were always other adults around as well as lifeguards, so she knew we were safe. And she had things to do. It wasn't easy to get things done with a houseful of kids.

My parents teamed up to do something similar on Sundays when we were growing up. They would drop all of us kids off at church and then go back home together. They would always laugh and say they were going home to "read *The Chicago Tribune*." I imagine they really wanted some time alone together and that was the only chance they were going to get all week.

Once again, I was put in charge. My parents would drop us at the curb in front of the church, and that's when I took over. I would usher the kids inside and get them seated, which because we always seemed to be running late, often meant sitting in the front row since those were the only spots left. Then I would make sure that everyone behaved during the service. In fact, I was always so concerned about what my brothers and sisters were doing that I hardly paid attention to the sermons at all. One time, when we were leaving church, the minister stopped me and said, "I talked about you today. Did you hear me?" I'd been so preoccupied with my siblings that I'd missed it entirely. My brother Jeff says the minister pointed to us there in the front row and held us up as an example. After all, we were such good kids to attend church every weekend even without our parents. We stopped going soon after that. I always thought it was because we moved, but my brother insists it's because Mom and Dad got wind of what the minister said, and after that, they were too embarrassed to bring us back!

WHEN I WAS STILL IN SCHOOL, my grandparents—my mom's parents—found out about a summer camp that was created specifically for kids with diabetes, and they arranged for me to go for a week. The idea behind the camp was to help kids learn how to live on their own with their condition. I hadn't been around a lot of kids with diabetes at that point in my life, so it was really an education.

The place was officially named Camp Hendon, after Dr. James Robert Hendon, who was the first endocrinologist in the state of Kentucky, but everyone there called it Camp Hope. All the kids slept in tents, and my tentmate—her name was Joy (Joy at Camp Hope!)—was a very different kind of kid than I was. She could hardly do anything for herself. She couldn't give herself shots. She couldn't go to sleep without being told a story, so I had to tell her one every night. The counselors were really appreciative of how I took care of her because they didn't have time to give her all the extra attention she needed. It was like I was her babysitter, only she wasn't that much younger than I was. I remember thinking, *Come on, Joy, grow up and get it together*. I even said something like that to her, though the words I chose were a bit more encouraging than that. I told her what my parents had always told me, that she could do these things for herself and that she didn't need me, or anyone else, to do them for her.

The experience made me appreciate how my parents had handled my diabetes. They always treated me like I was capable and trustworthy, and even if that bothered me sometimes, when I got to Camp Hendon, the alternative suddenly looked a whole lot worse. I saw Joy as someone to be pitied, and I definitely didn't want that to be me.

That isn't to say that everything about managing my diabetes came easily to me. Food was something I struggled with for much of my life, starting when I was very young. I was always extremely skinny as a kid. At one point, when I was about six years old, I was significantly underweight. It led to recurring tensions in our house, particularly with my mom. No one ever made a big deal about the shots I had to take for my diabetes, but when the doctor put me on appetite stimulants, that was a big deal. My mother would fuss at me for needing them and would continually try to get me to eat things I didn't want or like. I hated eggs, for example, but I had to eat two of them every morning for breakfast because that's what my dad ate. From her point of view, he seemed to be in pretty good shape, so if eggs worked for him, they ought to work for me. I had to finish those eggs before I could leave for school or I would catch hell. Sometimes the standoffs with Mom would go on so long that I would be late for school, which I didn't like. Often, I would wolf them down, trying to ignore the taste that I hated so much, but pretty soon, I figured out how to hide them.

We had this old farmhouse table in the kitchen, where we

always ate breakfast. It was a round wooden table with a big base that had ledges built into it. When I didn't like something, I would wait until Mom wasn't looking and hide it in one of those ledges. It wasn't just me, either. All the kids learned how to do it. Of course, Mom found the food eventually, and I got into trouble. After that, I had no choice but to finish my eggs.

I knew Mom was concerned about my eating for good reason, but at the time it seemed to me like I had enough to deal with and that maybe it wouldn't have killed her to offer me something else to eat once in a while. Day after day, I had to swallow these things that I really didn't like. It never occurred to me then that she might not have known how to handle it all. Back then, information about diabetes was a lot harder to come by. You couldn't just look things up on the internet or go to Amazon to buy a book with suitable recipes. She knew what worked for my dad, so that's what she trusted to work for me. It probably wasn't an area where she felt like she could afford to experiment.

To be fair, Mom made more of an effort than I gave her credit for at the time. For example, I couldn't have cake for my birthday, of course, even though that's what most kids got, so she would cut up a watermelon into a pile of melon balls so I could still have something special. (Despite the fact that it has natural sugar, I was always allowed fruit, just not too much of it.) And Mom must have been doing something right because my blood sugar was generally well controlled when I was a kid. In addition to monitoring what I ate, she also advocated exercise and was insistent that all of us kids walk to and from school each day. School wasn't just around the corner either. It was a forty-five-minute walk each way. But it was her way of making sure we got regular exercise. Even when it rained, she wouldn't drive us. She just made sure we were bundled up in our raincoats and rain boots, and then she sent us on our way. Being from Swedish stock, she never thought bad weather was a reason to stay inside.

My siblings and I walked together to elementary school until I graduated to junior high. At that point, I started walking by myself. I was in eighth grade when I discovered there was a drugstore on my route. I often had pocket money from babysitting, so I would stop at the drugstore on the way home and spend it on candy, the kind of stuff Mom never let me have, like Butterfinger bars and Bit-O-Honey taffy. Oh, how I loved Bit-O-Honey. Nobody knew because I always finished it before I got home. Not my parents. Not my siblings. Nobody but the drugstore owner. I got my insulin from that same drugstore, but if he made that connection, he never said anything. It was my secret rebellion. Mom and Dad never checked my blood sugar. That was my job, just like giving myself shots, so they never caught on.

Testing my blood sugar was something I had to do so often that I got pretty good at it. I admit, however, that I sometimes wouldn't test so I didn't have to know if it was out of the normal range. I imagine my blood sugar could get pretty high back then after I ate my secret candy bars, but I figured as long as I was able to function, it was fine. And I was functioning.

At least that's what I thought. Mom remembers one time when I was in junior high that I didn't come home from school when she was expecting me. She waited and waited, and just when she was starting to really worry, I finally walked in the door. I apparently burst into tears right then and there. I told her I had gotten confused and couldn't find my way home. That kind of confusion is more a symptom of low blood sugar rather than high (so I probably can't blame that one on the candy), but maybe I wasn't always as in control as I felt like I was. Still to this day, I have no memory of that happening, though my mom sure does.

Sneaking those candy bars was something I always felt bad about. I felt bad about eating them, and I felt bad about hiding it from everyone, especially my mom. Despite that, I continued to do it for at least a year. It's the first time that I remember thinking about myself as a "bad diabetic." I felt like I was "bad" because I was violating what my dad always referred to as "the rules" of having diabetes.

"Bad diabetic" is a term I've often heard people use over the years to describe someone who struggles with their diabetes or has suffered negative outcomes as a result. But it's a term I've grown to hate. After all, everyone has struggles. Everyone has bad things happen to them, sometimes through no fault of their own and sometimes the opposite. There seems to be a view among some people that individuals with diabetes are supposed to be perfect in terms of their diet, exercise, and lifestyle habits, but that's an impossible expectation. Nobody is perfect all the time. Everyone makes mistakes and falls short now and then. Everyone has good days and bad ones, but that doesn't make them bad people if something goes wrong. It took me years to realize that that way of thinking really isn't fair, and it doesn't help people move forward with their lives in healthy and productive ways.

At the time, I always thought of myself as a bad diabetic whenever I failed to make the best choices. But what teenager makes good choices all the time? (If we're being honest, what adult makes good choices all the time?) I had spent my whole life being told what the rules were, especially what the rules were around what I could and couldn't eat. Food battles with my mom were a regular part of my childhood, so it's not all that surprising that the first real attempts I made to exert control over my life had to do with food. Kids do a lot of different stuff at that age to assert their independence. My rebellion just happened to revolve not around drugs or who I dated or what I wore but around candy bars.

Looking back now, I wish I hadn't been so hard on myself. Yes, I indulged in some secret treats that maybe weren't the best choices I could have made, but they weren't the worst ones either. For one thing, I never ended up sick or in the hospital as a result. It was hard on my self-esteem to think of myself as someone who was "bad" when, really, I was just acting like a normal kid.

I also didn't spend nearly as much time thinking of myself as a "good diabetic," even though there are lots of examples that would have counted in the good column. I was good about taking my shots. I was good about getting exercise. I was good at taking care of my siblings. I was, by and large, a good daughter, a good sister, a good student, and a good person. When I was at camp, I felt like I was excellent at managing my diabetes compared to my tentmate, Joy, who could hardly do anything for herself. When my family was living in Columbia, Missouri, I was so good and my blood sugar was so consistent that the doctors wanted to put me in a controlled situation so they could study me. I spent about a month in the hospital that summer as they tried to figure out what was working so well. (I'm not sure if they ever came up with any answers.) There were other kids there, too, a group of about five of us with a variety of conditions that were being monitored. There wasn't a lot to do, and I remember that we had wheelchair races to pass the time. The nurses would task us with folding diapers to keep us busy. One of the other kids, a young boy, ended up dying that summer. I don't know what his condition was (it wasn't diabetes), but I do remember he bled through his skin. No one ever explained to us what happened, but all of us were pretty upset about it.

WHEN I WASN'T THINKING OF MYSELF as a bad diabetic, most of the time I considered myself a pretty normal kid dealing with pretty normal kid stuff. I spent the first decade of my life in Wichita, but after that, we had to move every couple of years as Dad climbed steadily up the corporate ladder at Sears and Roebuck and took on new roles. After our move from Wichita to Columbia when I was ten, we went to Kansas City, Kansas, when I was twelve. That was a tough year for me.

In Columbia, we had lived in a neighborhood with a bunch of kids that my siblings and I liked to hang around with. In the evenings, we would gather outside and play things like four square, kick the can, or dodgeball. Our family always ate later than every-body else, so the neighborhood kids would slowly start gathering in our yard after dinner, waiting for the Henderson kids to finish. They needed us to make teams. There were five of us, after all, enough to make up the numbers.

When we moved to Kansas City, everything was different, and I felt isolated without my old friends. I had always been a good student, but that year my teacher, Mrs. Dummit, decided she didn't like the slant of my handwriting. I was left-handed, so my writing slanted in the opposite direction from everyone else's. It had never been a problem before, but suddenly Mrs. Dummit was giving me an F on all my papers just because of my hand-writing. Then she'd make me rewrite them in the opposite slant, which was not easy to do, and return them to her the next day. For some reason, she had this idea that everyone's writing should look the same. I felt humiliated, like I was being singled out for no good reason (which even with the benefit of hindsight still feels true!). It shook my world because I'd always been told I was a good student, and it made me think that maybe I wasn't so good after all. That experience is probably a big reason why I still make a point of avoiding a cookie-cutter mindset where everyone has to be the same and instead try to appreciate people's differences.

To make matters worse, two streets away lived a girl named Sally. She was the same age as me but a lot bigger. I was always this skinny, gangly kid, so most of my classmates were bigger than me, but only Sally thought that meant it was OK to bully me. That was also the year that President John F. Kennedy was shot, which was a big deal to just about everyone at the time. I wasn't old enough to really understand politics, but I remember getting home that day to find my mom lying in bed crying. She had never been one to show a lot of emotion, so it shook me up to see her like that. It was another thing we didn't really talk about, so I didn't fully understand what was happening at the time.

All in all, it was an awful year. I would often cry myself to sleep at night. But I would also make myself a promise. I would repeat over and over to myself that next year I would be the most popular girl in my grade. Next year I would be the most popular girl in my grade. I said it so often that I started to believe it.

And it actually worked! The following summer we moved again, this time to Park Ridge, Illinois, just outside of Chicago, and there I became popular. No one bullied me. There were no teachers who gave me a hard time. In fact, just about everyone seemed to like me. I had lots of friends, even a few that my parents didn't entirely approve of.

Sadly, however, my triumph was short-lived because we had to move yet again about a year later. Still, the experience gave me a sense of power in a world where it felt like so much was outside my control. I took it as proof that I could affect my own destiny even in the face of adversity. If I just focused on what I wanted, perhaps I was capable of willing it so.

Chapter 3

INDEPENDENCE

WE MOVED ONLY ONCE MORE after Park Ridge, this time to Louisville, Kentucky, where my family finally got to stay put for a while. After five cities in a handful of years, Dad's job no longer required him to move every year or two to take on a new role, so Louisville is where I stayed until graduating from high school.

By the time that happened, I was ready for a change. As I wrote before, my parents had gone to Lake Forest College outside Chicago, which is also where a lot of Mom's family went, but I wanted something different, something of my own. When it was my time to go away to school, I chose the University of Missouri in Columbia, a place where I'd had some of my happiest times growing up. And because I'd always been told by my teachers that I could write well, I decided to study journalism.

At the time, the University of Missouri was featured on *Playboy*'s list of the top ten party schools in the country, and once I arrived, I had no intention of letting their ranking drop. By the time I left home, I was more than ready to live life on my own terms, to do what I wanted to do, and to make my own rules for a change. I was the first to arrive at every party and every kegger. If my friends were having a drink, I would have two. I ate what I wanted, and I would go days without checking my blood sugar. Life was totally different than it had been when I was growing up, and I quickly found that I loved it that way.

Just like my dad before me, I guarded my privacy fiercely, which meant I was truly handling my diabetes on my own for the first time in my life. Even though I felt like it had always been my responsibility growing up, I always had Mom and Dad as backup, and I went to the doctor regularly. When I went off to college, there weren't any endocrinologists around—not that I was looking all that hard for one. I didn't talk with any of my friends about my condition. I lived in a dorm at first and then in a sorority house after pledging Chi Omega, and I was able to keep my insulin in my own mini fridge next to my bed. One of my sorority sisters was studying to become a nurse, and she might have picked up on things, but we never talked openly about it. Growing up, I had shared a room with my sister Cindy, who was used to seeing me give myself shots, but now I was doing it all in secret. I never took my diabetes supplies out in front of anyone. Never.

My mom says that because I had always been so capable, she wasn't worried about me when I left home. Besides, I'd been adamant about going several hundred miles away to college, so she figured there wasn't much she could do anyway. She did get reports from time to time from her younger sister living in Kansas City, Missouri, whom I would stay with on occasion. Apparently, her sister told her that I "ran a little wild" because I would often stay out late when I was visiting her, but my mom trusted me enough to let me figure things out on my own.

I suppose I was like a typical college student in that way, testing my boundaries, enjoying my freedom, and yes, maybe even getting a little wild sometimes. But for the most part, I functioned pretty well, so I figured I didn't have much to worry about. After all, I kept up my grades, and I held down a part-time job. Of course, my part-time job was working as a waitress in a campus bar, which maybe wasn't the best choice for me. My boyfriend at the time was the bartender, and he wasn't such a good influence either. Still, none of us drank much on the job. By the end of the night, you could smell the stuff on you, in your clothes and clinging to your hair, so it wasn't all that appealing. In fact, I'd often ask for just an orange juice at the end of my shift. Outside of work, of course, was a very different story.

Still, despite discovering alcohol and becoming lax about my blood sugar monitoring, I never reached a point where I got really sick. Once a year or so I would find myself feeling pretty worn out, so without telling anyone, I would go to the hospital to get rebalanced. I would usually stay for a few days while they monitored my blood sugar and made sure I was well hydrated since dehydration is common among people with diabetes. I didn't think it was such a big deal—after all, I had been in the hospital plenty of times growing up—but I remember once a doctor giving me a good talking to. He said to me: "If you don't improve the way you're handling your diabetes, you won't make it to thirty."

To my ears now, it sounds like a stark warning, but I brushed it off then. I don't think I really believed him. After all, my dad drank regularly and worked hard, and he had already lived well past thirty. Or maybe I just didn't care. I sort of figured that if I was only going to live to thirty, then I was going to have a hell of a time until then.

THAT'S PRETTY MUCH THE STATE I WAS IN when I met David, my future husband. The way he remembers it, he admired me from afar since our freshman year. The first time he asked me out was in September of our senior year, but I blew him off, telling him that I preferred older guys and that I was headed to Europe for the summer after I graduated, so dating wasn't a priority anyway. It was true: I was saving up from my waitressing job so I could go on a big trip that my friends and I were planning. To me, nothing was a bigger deal than that trip.

I would see David around, but that was basically it between us until toward the end of the school year when, one night, a bunch of us were at a bar called Harpo's. One of my friends was dating one of David's friends, so she knew that he liked me, and she told me so. Then, well, I got very drunk that night and said to him, "David Novak, when are you going to get the balls to ask me out?" I never was a quiet drunk.

I think I shocked him a little, but he thought quickly on his feet. "Um, uh, um, how about tomorrow night?"

He was majoring in journalism too, so we decided to go to a journalism party together the next night. David still remembers that I was wearing a gray fuzzy sweater that was one of my favorites. He was driving, and we got lost on our way to the party. So we gave up looking and spent the whole night talking. It may not have been love at first sight for us, but it was love at first date. From then on, that was it. We were inseparable. About four weeks later, at our graduation ceremony, we walked down the aisle together to get our degrees, and he told his family afterward that the gal he'd been walking with was the gal he was going to marry. Of course, he didn't tell me that, not yet anyway, but they all knew.

After graduation, I went home to stay with my parents for a while before I headed to Europe. After about a week, David showed up at the house. He told my parents, who had only met him briefly at the graduation ceremony, that he was on his way home to his parents' place and that he just wanted to stop in and see me. He only meant to come for the day, but then I asked if he could stay for a few nights. My parents agreed, and so did he.

It wasn't the best timing because I'd just had a couple of wisdom teeth pulled, but I was excited to see him, so I rallied, and the two of us went out that night. By the time we got home, my parents were already in bed. I wasn't feeling too hot—I think I had developed a bit of an infection—and David was concerned enough that he actually went into my parents' bedroom to wake up my mom. It was around 11 p.m. when he said to her, "Mrs. Henderson, Wendy's not feeling very well. I think you better go check on her."

So she did. Her primary concern was that I was having trouble with my blood sugar—and so that's how David learned that I had diabetes. He probably had an inkling before that, but he hadn't asked too many questions. Love is so often blind, after all. Thankfully, my blood sugar was stable; I was just aching from my teeth. So, Mom got me an aspirin and headed back to bed. As she walked down the hallway, she passed the room where David was staying. The door was open, and she saw him sitting on the bed wringing his hands. He was that worried about me.

During my time in college, a couple different guys had come to visit me at my parents' house. Mom had liked one of them OK, but she thought the other was kind of a jerk. But when she saw David sitting there like that, she thought, *That's the guy for Wendy.* She could tell that he really cared about me.

I hope I made as good a first impression on David's parents. Before my trip to Europe, I went to visit him at his parents' house for a few days in Gaithersburg, Maryland, outside of Washington, DC I fell in love with his family right away.

David was close with his parents and both of his younger sisters, Karen and Susan, and they were all so affectionate with one another. I called them "cling-ons" because they would all get on the sofa together in the evenings and sort of cling on to each other. It was like they were covered in glue, and they just stuck. His dad had been a surveyor for the federal government, which meant they spent much of David's childhood on the move, living out of trailers, the biggest being only about eight feet wide by forty-six feet long. That meant they were used to packing into small spaces together, and even when they eventually moved into a house with more space, the habit stuck. They were very open with one another, too, and really talked about things. I loved everything about them.

The first time David hinted about getting married, I didn't take him seriously. I was going to Europe come hell or high water, and he'd known that since the first time we met. Marriage didn't fit into the picture. But one night, while I was staying at his parents' house, David and I were going somewhere together in his white Chevy Monte Carlo with its black top (he really loved that car), and he brought up the subject again. I took him seriously that time. I just had this feeling in my gut telling me that he was a really good guy. He was serious about me, so I figured I had better be serious too. I said to him, "You know, I would love to marry you, but I probably won't live to see forty, and I probably won't be able to have children."

David knew I had diabetes, of course, but I didn't think he understood the possible effects. I figured it was only fair to spell it out for him. What I thought was this big revelation turned out to be not such a big deal after all.

He just said, "It doesn't matter. All I want is you." And that was that.

It was just a day or two later, while we were watching Johnny Carson one night in his parents' living room, that he got down on his knee in front of the chair where I was sitting, and he proposed. It had been only about eight weeks since we started dating, and in just a few days I was headed off to Europe for two months. Still, it felt right, so I didn't hesitate. I said yes.

I MAY HAVE SAID YES to the proposal, but I still had every intention of going to Europe. Nothing could deter me from that. I think it was that sick room with all the travel posters on the walls that made me want to go so badly. On my itinerary were places I had dreamed about for a long time. There were two other senior girls in my sorority who were planning postgraduation trips, so we decided to go together. It was the three of us: Jeannie Jacoby, Miriam Kiely, and me.

Miriam was short with beautiful long blonde hair and big green eyes. Jeannie was tall, nearly six feet tall, with dark hair and dark eyes. We were all just twenty-one years old, and the three of us got a lot of attention running around Europe together. Jeannie, in fact, stopped traffic once while she was crossing the street in Italy.

When I got on the plane, I turned to my friends and said, "I have some news for you guys. I think I'm getting married!"

"Really? To whom?" That was their first reaction. David and I had been dating for such a short time, they couldn't imagine who I was talking about. Once I told them the story, though, they were happy for me.

We flew into London with just enough money to spend two months traveling around Europe as long as we stayed in hostels and cheap hotels. After London, we went to Paris, Amsterdam, Berlin, a couple different cities in Italy. It was a real education. I saw red light districts for the first time in Amsterdam and then again in Berlin. I went to my first lesbian bar in London. In Paris, we met a Frenchman with a plane who wanted to take us on a day trip to look at another plane in another city for some reason. Why he wanted to do this was never really clear, but we still said yes. We got on a small plane with two of his colleagues, both lawyers, and then the six of us went to look at some other plane, followed by a grand steak dinner at a restaurant (probably some of the best food we ate all trip) before flying back to Paris. Looking back now, I wonder if the whole thing was a little sketchy. The guy could have been running drugs for all we knew, but I loved it. I thought it was so neat flying on a small plane, being in a new place, and meeting new people. It was incredible. And he was a perfect gentleman. I guess he just thought it would be fun to have us along.

After nearly two months in Europe, we made it back to London a few days before we were due to return home. It was there, with just two days to go on our itinerary, that our money ran out. This was long before the days of cell phones and easy money transfers via Zelle or Venmo. We weren't even in regular touch with our parents during the trip—because calls were so expensive, we mostly wrote letters or postcards to people back home— so we had to figure out for ourselves what to do. We decided to go down to Carnaby Street in Soho, where there were lots of shops, and try to sell our blue jeans. This was 1974, and Levi's bell bottoms—which were, of course, what we had—were a hot ticket. We would hang around on the sidewalk until someone about our age would pass by, and then we'd ask them if they wanted to buy our jeans. Finally, a young woman agreed, and we made enough to get us through our last couple of days until we could go home.

All the while I traveled with my insulin. I didn't always have a refrigerator, so I just kept it in my backpack along with my needles. I didn't talk to my tripmates about it, and I didn't have any problems with my blood sugar on the trip. Of course, per usual at that time in my life, I didn't test myself very often either. I probably ran high a lot, but you can't always tell. You feel lows more easily than you do highs.

Symptoms of High Blood Sugar

High blood sugar, or hyperglycemia, often doesn't cause symptoms until blood glucose levels are significantly elevated. Food choices, exercise, illness, and medications can all contribute to high blood sugar levels in people with diabetes.

Early symptoms can include the following:

- Frequent urination
- Thirst
- Blurry vision
- Fatigue
- Headaches

If left untreated, it can lead to worsening hyperglycemia, dehydration, buildup of acid in the blood, and the development of ketones, which can cause the following symptoms:

- Fruity-smelling breath (due to ketones)
- Shortness of breath
- Dry mouth
- Weakness
- Nausea and vomiting
- Confusion
- Abdominal pain
- Coma

We returned from Europe in July. Both of my girlfriends were headed back to marry the guys they'd been dating in college, and I hoped I was too. But for a while there, I wasn't so sure.

I missed David like crazy, but it was a long time to be apart. We had only been dating for a couple of months when I left, and I was gone basically the same length of time, so I couldn't help but wonder if things might have changed while I was away. It didn't help that about halfway through the trip, I abruptly stopped getting letters from him.

I had given him my itinerary before I left, which included the addresses of where we'd be staying at each stop, and David had been sending letters to me at each place. I got lots of letters from him for about a month, and then, all of a sudden, there was nothing.

I didn't know what to think about that. When it was nearing time for us to come home, I wasn't sure what to do. Should I go to Washington, DC, near where his parents lived, to see him? Or should I return to Louisville, Kentucky, to my parents' house? Finally, I decided I had better call him to find out. His mother, Jean, answered when I called. David wasn't home at the time, so I told her my dilemma.

"David stopped writing to me. Has he got another girlfriend?" I asked her.

I've always thought that she could have gotten rid of me right then and there if she wanted to. She knew about my diabetes, after all, but she never said anything to me about it, so I didn't know what she thought. I learned later that when David told her, she simply said to him, "If you love her, then you've got to follow your heart." I've always been grateful to her for that because she had a hand in helping our relationship along. In that important moment, when I was doubting whether David and I truly had a future, she said to me, "Oh honey, you need to come to Washington because he really, really misses you." That was all I needed. As soon as I got back, I went straight to the Novaks' house.

It turned out that David had lost my mailing list, which is why the letters had suddenly stopped. He had called my mother to ask her for the list, but he says she wouldn't give it to him. She says she didn't have it. They still disagree about it to this day, and David jokingly says he's never forgiven her for it.

WHEN I GOT BACK INTO THE COUNTRY, my parents didn't even know right away because I was so happily entrenched with the Novaks. That may seem strange to some, especially now that everyone keeps in constant touch via cell phone and social media, but that's not how things were back then. If I wanted to talk to my family while I was away, I had to make a collect call, which you just didn't do very often because it was so expensive. Besides, my family was always very independent, so I stayed at the Novaks' for a while, living in their basement, until one day I called my mother on the phone. While I was talking with her, my father broke in on the conversation to tell me that I needed to get my ass out of that house! He thought that I had overstayed my welcome, so I figured it was time to find my own apartment.

Of course, both David and I needed to find jobs. We both looked like crazy for something in Washington, DC, but there was a recession going on, one that boasted an unusual combination of high inflation and high unemployment at the same time. The upshot was that no one was hiring unless you had experience, and we were fresh out of college. Neither of us had any big plan for what we wanted to do with our lives either. We just wanted something that paid decently so we could move forward with our lives.

While I was still in Europe, David had gotten a position at an ad agency, which he supplemented with a night job working the desk at a Holiday Inn. After I returned, I spent weeks looking for something and finally got a job selling classified ads in the advertising department at *Washingtonian* magazine. It was a hip, popular magazine that had been around for about a decade. I was the primary breadwinner back then because my job paid significantly better, but to be honest, neither of us were making very much. We were broke and barely making ends meet, but it was a start.

Just like my dad, I made a point of keeping my condition a secret from everyone at work. It may not have been quite as bad as in my dad's day, but there was still a stigma. Some people believed that an individual with diabetes would be sickly and miss a lot of work. Others worried about the symptoms you might display. The job market was already tough enough. I didn't need employers worrying about my medical condition on top of it. As best I could, I avoided giving myself an insulin shot at work, but when I had to do it, I would lock myself in a bathroom stall first. I was paranoid that someone would see my needle and think that I was a drug addict!

I liked my job at the *Washingtonian*, but I hated the commute. David and I had found an apartment about five minutes from his parents' house in Gaithersburg, and I had to travel from there all the way to downtown Washington each day. David would drive me in the mornings to Chevy Chase, Maryland, where his office was located, and then I would take the bus to L Street, not far from the White House. Traffic was always terrible, and it was at least an hour and a half each way. But we were in love, we were going to get married, and there was no stopping us.

About that apartment: I remember it as my apartment. David remembers it as his apartment. We were not living together, but we were both there all the time even though, technically, he was still living with his parents while I was living in the apartment. That was the official story anyway.

Of course, that setup couldn't last long, so David's mom finagled things to make sure we got married sooner rather than later. She insisted that we do it before the end of the year and suggested that Thanksgiving would be a good time.

When I told my dad I was getting married, he was busily reading the newspaper. After I relayed the news, he slowly lowered his paper and peered at me over his glasses. "You're really serious about this guy," he said, half asking, half reading the situation. I told him that I was. He took the news in stride after that. By that point, I think everybody understood that we really cared for each other.

We got married in November of 1974 in Louisville, Kentucky, where my parents lived. It was a small wedding at St. Matthews Presbyterian Church followed by a reception at my parents' house.

I'd never been to the church where we got married, but we chose it because the minister who married us, Dr. Mobley, had known me throughout high school. He'd been in charge of the youth group I attended at another church. David and I had to go in together to meet with him before he would marry us, and he asked us a bunch of questions about our future, like what values we shared and whether we planned to raise children in the church. David and I hadn't known each other long enough to have discussed much of this stuff, so it was probably a good thing for us to do. After all, we'd only been dating for a total of about seven months when we got married, and for two of those, we hadn't even been in the same country.

Still, I think that sometimes maybe it's better not to know too much. The older I get, the more I think that. Given where we were in our lives at the time and where we were in our still very new relationship, we never should have gotten married. Not on paper, at least. But we went ahead with the wedding anyway, and nearly fifty years later, I'm still so happy that we did.

Chapter 4

RISK AND REWARD

DURING THE MEETING DAVID AND I had with Dr. Mobley before the wedding, he told us something that always stuck with me. He said that in a marriage, it's like there are two people engaged in a dance. You dance together, of course, but you also have to dance alone sometimes. That means being able to give your partner space and freedom to do their own thing. When that happens, it doesn't mean your partner doesn't love you. In fact, your partner loves you just as much when you're apart as they do when you're together. It just means that, sometimes, each of us needs to dance alone.

He was trying to prepare us for the fact that, when you fall in love, you want to be together all the time, but marriage is different. I would often remind myself of his wisdom through the years when things got a little tough. The first time I remember thinking about it was when David would play tennis without me. We liked to play tennis together. In fact, one of our first dates had been on the tennis court where I lost a six-pack of Buckhorn beer to David when he beat me. But after we got married, sometimes he would go off on his own to play with a friend or colleague. When we were living in Gaithersburg, we had only the one car, his cherished white Monte Carlo with its black top, so when he went off to play tennis, I was stuck at home alone.

When that happened, I would tell myself that it was OK that he was off doing his own thing without me because that was him dancing his dance. Of course, I needed to be able to dance too. I never much liked the feeling of being stuck, so I decided to go out and buy myself a bike so that I could go places when David had the car. I went to Sears and Roebuck, of course, because that's where Dad worked, and I bought a Free Spirit bicycle with a basket on the front. Then when David was out on his own, I would use it to go out on my own.

It wasn't a perfect solution, mostly because of all the times I got into a wreck on that bicycle. I often carried this big pink bag with me, which I would fill up with stuff when I went shopping, and then, on the way back home, it would get caught in the wheels. I never seriously hurt myself, just scraped myself up here and there, and it never stopped me from using that bike. So while it wasn't the perfect solution, it worked well enough.

David and I got married so quickly and at such a young age that I'm not sure that either of us had any real sense of what marriage would actually be like, so we had to figure it out together. One pattern that we adopted early on was something that I had grown accustomed to in childhood: moving. David had had a similar experience growing up. His dad, Charles, as I described earlier, was a surveyor for the US government, traveling the country to measure unmapped regions, so just like me, David was used to moving from place to place to accommodate his father's job.

Perhaps because of that shared history, we didn't resist the idea of moving frequently for work. We spent less than two years in Gaithersburg before we started thinking about moving on. Both of us felt like our jobs were dead ends, so I suggested we look outside the DC area for something new. David wrote fifty letters to the top fifty ad agencies across the country, and the first one to respond was Ketchum, MacLeod & Grove in Pittsburgh, Pennsylvania. He went up there to interview and got offered a job at twice his previous salary. We had to take it, so I followed him there and got a job at the same company, working on the PR side of things while he worked in advertising.

Working together was a bit of a struggle, at least for me. At the *Washingtonian*, I had been the top salesperson, but at Ketchum, I always felt like I was comparing myself to David even though we did very different things. And he was successful at his job as an advertising account executive, whereas I didn't enjoy PR nearly as much as I had enjoyed being in sales. It wasn't long before David, too, felt like his opportunities in Pittsburgh were limited. He wanted to grow his career, take on bigger accounts, so once again I suggested we start looking elsewhere. I said to him, "If we can't find new jobs within a year, let's just move. After all, we can go anywhere."

After only three years in Pittsburgh, David got offered a job in Dallas, so we up and moved again. He landed at the ad agency

Tracy-Locke, working as an account executive for Frito-Lay accounts, which was a big step up from what he had been doing. Pretty soon I got a job too, selling TV time for the ABC affiliate WFAA. I felt like I was finally in a job that I really loved. I got to wine and dine clients, who were typically business owners and executives, taking them out to lunch or dinner and selling them advertising packages. I even put commercials together for some of the local businesses that didn't have the experience to do it themselves. I was there for four years and ended up rising to a senior position before it all came to a screeching halt. I had to leave the job abruptly because, after eight years of marriage, I got pregnant.

I DON'T REMEMBER EVER TALKING with my parents or doctor growing up about how diabetes might affect my ability to have a baby. I must have known something about it because I told David before we got married that he needed to prepare for the fact that it might never happen.

My mom remembers getting a book out of the library about diabetes soon after I was diagnosed so she could learn more about the condition. There was one passage in the book that really concerned her about how many women with diabetes are unable to have children. She says it was something she worried about because she knew what a good mother I would be based on how nurturing I was with my younger siblings. Whether she decided it was best not to pass those concerns on to me or I just blocked it out after she did, I don't think I'll ever know for sure. All I know is that at some point I started to believe that having a baby might be a possibility after all.

At the age of thirty, I decided I wanted to try. At that point in my life, I'd never had any really big problems with my blood sugar. I'd had times here and there when I felt run-down and went to the doctor or the hospital to sort things out, but I'd always felt like I was pretty stable and healthy overall. The first time I talked to a doctor about the idea of getting pregnant, I was told it would be risky. After that, I essentially went doctor shopping until I found an endocrinologist who was willing to work through the risks with me. He gave me the go-ahead to give it a shot.

I hadn't even floated the idea by David yet. I went home that night and said to him, "Hey, I want to have a baby." His response was one of disbelief. He didn't know what I was talking about. After all, I had told him from the start that we wouldn't be having children.

"But you can't have a baby," he said to me. I told him what my new doctor had said, and David figured, if the doctor said it was OK, then it must be OK. We decided to start trying right away. After all, we had waited this long. There was no time to waste.

If your blood sugar isn't under control, it can make pregnancy more difficult at every stage, and that includes conception, so when I didn't get pregnant right away, I was immediately upset. After trying for just one month, I decided that David needed to get his fertility checked in case it was him and not me, so I sent him off to a clinic. The doctor there told him he was more than ready to father a child, which only made me more nervous that it was me. As it turned out, I didn't need to worry so much. It was only about a month later—so two months of trying, which, as most doctors will tell you, is not much time at all—that I went back to my endocrinologist, who congratulated me on being pregnant.

Later that same evening, I called Mom to tell her the news. Her response was, "Oh honey, I'm sorry." It was the last thing I wanted to hear. At first, it shocked me because I hadn't expected that reaction. I never believed that pregnancy was going to impact my health, so I had gone ahead and planned the whole thing without talking to her about it. She obviously had a different perspective. She was concerned that I was putting myself at risk.

It turned out that her concerns were valid. I had no idea what I was getting into when I got pregnant—or maybe I didn't want to know—but in just three weeks, I went from having normal vision to barely being able to see. I had developed diabetic retinopathy, which is when the retina of the eye becomes damaged. It's a complication that can happen to people with diabetes, especially in pregnancy. In my case, all these blood vessels suddenly grew in my eyes, which then leaked and clouded my vision quite badly.

When I went to see my endocrinologist, he took one look at me and said, "Oh my God, I don't even recognize your eyes." He sent me straight from his office to the eye doctor. I guess it didn't occur to anyone to suggest that I call someone for a ride, so I drove myself. I had driven myself to the endocrinologist's office, after all, so I guess it seemed OK. But on my way to the eye doctor, I hit a "Men at Work" sign, which caused all the actual men at work to go running in different directions. Everyone was OK, thank goodness, but I wouldn't be driving again for a while.

After that, I had to go to an ophthalmologist for laser

treatments about three times a week throughout my entire pregnancy. Blood would seep out of those vessels in my eyes, and then the doctors would laser them dry. Even then, it would take time to regain my sight afterward because the body had to clear away the blood. When it got bad, it was like I was looking through several sheets of wax paper.

The effect would come and go, so at one point, I invented a sort of game to play with myself in the mornings. When I woke up, I would look in the direction of the light switch on the wall. If I could see it, then it was going to be a good day. If I couldn't see it, then it was going to be tougher.

When it got to the point where I couldn't see the big E on the eye chart, I knew I was in trouble. That was when I had to have the first of my vitrectomies, two in each eye, where doctors go in surgically to remove the vitreous humor gel in the eye and then cut and seal off the blood vessels causing the damage.

The problem continued to get worse, and I could see progressively less and less over time. I was told there was a possibility that I would never get my vision back, but I always had this feeling that in the end, it was going to be OK. I don't have any explanation for that, but there was something in me that simply believed that I would be alright. That ability to believe in a positive outcome even when things look bleak is something I first started to develop in school when I was struggling (and just knew that I could become popular one day if I tried!). My eyesight wasn't the only reason I would need to call on that ability in the coming months. My sight was the first thing to go wrong, but it was hardly the only issue I faced during what turned out to be an eventful (to put it nicely) pregnancy.

Pregnancy and Diabetes

Despite the complications I experienced, people with diabetes can have healthy pregnancies. Here are some things to keep in mind that can help:

- If possible, prepare early. Doctors often recommend that your blood sugar levels are well managed for several months before becoming pregnant.

- Review your medications. Some medications that are otherwise safe are not safe to use while pregnant, so make sure to review what you're taking with your doctor.

- Be aware of changes in your insulin requirements. Your needs may change throughout your pregnancy, so be prepared to monitor and make changes when necessary.

- Know the risks. People with diabetes are at greater risk for things like preeclampsia, which I experienced, but many of these risks can be treated successfully. Ask your doctor about symptoms to watch out for, and make sure to have checkups regularly.

A FEW MONTHS INTO THE PREGNANCY, David was in the other room playing with our golden retriever, Brandy, when he suddenly heard this unbelievable sound coming from the next room. He came in and found me lying flat on my back. I had completely passed out. I was snoring—and I mean really snoring—in a way he had never heard before. He tried to rouse me, but I wouldn't wake up.

David called an ambulance. That was the first time in our relationship that we had to go to the hospital together. There I was diagnosed with toxemia, or what's often called preeclampsia, which can cause dangerously high blood pressure and problems with your kidneys. It can be a serious, even life-threatening condition, and doctors will often induce labor when it happens. I wasn't far enough along for that to happen, however, so instead I was told I would have to be on bed rest for the rest of my pregnancy —the whole remaining five months.

That wasn't the end of it either. I was told the placenta was too mature, which meant that the baby was in danger of not getting enough nutrients. To compensate, I had to eat huge steaks to boost my iron. Between that and not being allowed to move much from my bed, I kept gaining weight, which also is not uncommon for mothers with diabetes. I had gained a total of seventy-two pounds by the end of it. I had always been a fairly petite person, so seventy-two pounds was a lot. In fact, it represented about 60 percent of my original body weight!

At one point, I gained so much weight that when I rolled over in bed, I threw my back out. I couldn't believe it. I called myself "the ever-expanding woman." (David gave me an "endearing" nickname of his own, one which I'd rather not repeat.) I would just lie there in bed and grow and grow and grow. It felt like an out-of-body experience.

David was a trooper through all of it. I had never been so amazed by a guy in my life. I didn't even know that all this stuff could happen, so he was really caught by surprise. I had left my job when I got pregnant, so not only was David the only one working, but he also did all the grocery shopping, the laundry, and the cleaning. I hated being in bed all the time with nothing to do. That was when I invented the game with the light switch. If it was a day when I could see, at least I could read. When I couldn't see, things could get pretty hard.

David did get some help, however. Volunteers from an organization called Lighthouse for the Blind came by. They showed me how to organize things so I knew where they were when my sight was failing. They marked the light switches and other appliances with tape so I could control them by feel.

There was nothing else to do but live with it and adjust, so that's what I did. I even stopped drinking. I had been a big drinker ever since college, having at least one drink every night, just like my dad. One of the things that helped me stop was the Alcoholics Anonymous book on tape that the Lighthouse for the Blind brought me to listen to. I don't know how they knew that I could use a book like that, but it sure did help, at least through the duration of the pregnancy. I did my best to eat well and stay as healthy as possible, too, given my bedridden circumstances. The last thing I wanted to be during that time was a "bad diabetic," so I did everything I could. I even wore an early version of a portable insulin pump, which back then was heavy and cumbersome, the size of a phone book, with a steel needle that just plain hurt. But I didn't complain because I wanted my baby to have the best possible chance, and I believed that I could give that to her even with everything that was going wrong around me.

WE HAD A SCARE ABOUT TWENTY WEEKS before the due date when it looked like the baby might be coming very, very early. We were relieved when that didn't happen, but not for long. About ten weeks later, at ten weeks premature, our daughter Ashley was born.

I was already in the hospital when it started. I was having an amniocentesis to check on the state of the baby, and I thought the doctors must have hit her with that long needle they use because she immediately started going crazy. She was kicking and moving about, and pretty soon, I started having labor pains. The nurses went into a panic. I remember sitting there watching them, and it was like this shade was being drawn over my eyes. I could barely see a thing. I think my blood pressure must have spiked, and all this fluid started pumping into my eyes.

I didn't even have time to think after that. All of a sudden, they were putting me under so they could do an emergency C-section. One of the nurses was counting down, as they do when they're waiting for the anesthesia to kick in, when the anesthesiologist started to say, "Oh my God, if she's . . ." And that was the last thing

I heard. I never did find out what he was so concerned about, but it wasn't the most relaxing way to go into emergency surgery.

Meanwhile, someone called David at work. They pulled him out of a meeting to tell him I was in labor, and all he could think was, *She's not ready yet*. He was right. We weren't ready, but ready or not, it was happening, and it was happening fast.

When Ashley arrived, she weighed only four pounds, ten ounces. David got to see her first because I still hadn't come out of the anesthesia. When he arrived at the hospital, the doctor wrote down on a blackboard all the things that could go wrong with a baby that arrived as early as she had. He said that she could have trouble with her lungs, her heart, and her brain, but he also said that they just weren't sure yet. They would have to monitor her for a while, and we would have to wait and see. Then he asked if David wanted to see her.

David didn't know what to expect when he went down to the neonatal intensive care unit (NICU). He remembers there being all these tubes sticking out of Ashley, and her complexion was beet red. Even so, he thought she was the most beautiful thing he had ever seen. He reached his hand down to touch her, and right away she took his finger and squeezed it. He couldn't believe it. In that moment he knew in his heart that she was going to be OK. He was so confident of that fact that he started telling everyone that his baby girl was going to live.

After that, he came up to see me. He wanted to take me to see the baby, but I didn't want to go. I'd been told there was less than a 50 percent chance that she would make it, and I was afraid. I was afraid of what could happen. I was afraid of getting attached only to lose her. I just couldn't bear the thought of it. Meanwhile, David was walking around like a proud peacock talking about how beautiful the baby was, but I couldn't share his confidence that everything was going to be OK—at least not yet.

David kept reassuring me, telling me how strong she was already, how he could feel it when she'd grabbed his finger. Eventually, I felt ready to see her for myself, so he took me down to the NICU. I saw immediately that he was right about one thing at least: she really was a beautiful baby.

The doctors told us later that she didn't have any of the signs of being carried by a mother with diabetes. All the complications were a result of her coming so early, not my diabetes. I was very proud of that and took a lot of comfort from it. I had worked really hard to stay in control of my diabetes during that time, and at least I had given her the best chance that I could.

THE NEXT SEVERAL WEEKS were kind of a blur, but I remember spending a lot of time in the NICU. When the doctors got a chance to examine Ashley fully, they discovered that her lungs weren't fully developed. She had something called hyaline membrane disease, which is what John and Jackie Kennedy's premature baby had died of in the 1960s. There was talk of some valve in her heart that had to close, and if it didn't, she wouldn't make it. Otherwise, she appeared to be in decent shape, and they said she had a fighting chance.

David fell in love with the nurses there in the NICU. It didn't hurt that they were very good looking, but it was really more about how competent they were and how much they cared about their tiny charges. There were two in particular who, anytime a buzzer would go off, would jump right on it. We'd watch as they would turn babies over and pat them on the bottom just to get them breathing again. They were expert at it, and they handled these life-and-death situations like they were no big deal. It was amazing to see them work, and we felt like we were in really good hands.

Early on David asked them if there was anything special we could do that could help Ashley and give her a better chance. They said babies love to hear your voice, so when we couldn't be there to talk to her in person, we made audio tapes—cassettes at the time—talking to her about what had happened that day and how much we loved her. The nurses would play those tapes when we couldn't be there in person. They also told us that the first color babies see is red, so David went straight out to buy her a plastic red apple toy, the size of a mini basketball, with a big happy face on it. It was his first gift to her, and we always put her to bed with it. Ashley still has that apple, in fact, and has passed it on to her own children.

Slowly, things began to get better. In the NICU, the sickest infants were placed in the back, nearest the nurses' station, while the healthiest ones were placed up front. Ashley gradually made her way forward as she put on weight and her vitals improved. One of the surest signs of progress was when the nurses started teaching us how to care for her so we'd be prepared when it was time to take her home. One day, one of the neonatal nurses was showing me how to diaper Ashley—which was no easy feat given how small she was—and David kind of got in between us, swung his hips, and bumped me out of the way. "I can do this," he said. I laughed. I knew then and there that he was going to be a real hands-on father.

We had our bright moments in that NICU, but it was also hard. I remember one Sunday when a patient and a couple of babies got to go home. They always threw these big celebrations when babies got to leave the NICU because it was a big deal. I remember the doctor catching my eye then. I was trying my best to be happy for this other family, but he could tell I was devastated that Ash still didn't get to go home. He came around, gave me a hug, and patted my hands. "It's going to be OK," he told me. "We're gonna make it through this." I'll never forget that moment of kindness. It was enough to help me hold on a little longer. And he was right. We did make it through.

The goal was to get Ashley to five pounds, and then the doctors would discharge her. It took nearly a month, but she finally got there. We got word that they were sending her home.

Before that could happen, however, we needed some clothes for her. She'd only ever worn diapers and hospital blankets at that point, and we needed something we could take her home in. The problem was there weren't any places around that made clothes for preemies back then. Everything we could find was way too big, so we had the brilliant idea of going to Toys "R" Us to find doll clothes that could work. We found a doll about the same size as Ashley, bought it, and then removed its clothes. And it worked. They fit her perfectly.

There was just one final hiccup before we could finally get our little girl home, albeit a small one. Ashley had only ever been in the NICU, which was a highly controlled and sterile environment. Before we left, the nurses warned us, "When people see a new baby, it's natural for them to want to stop and have a look, to fawn over her a little, but don't let them do that with Ashley." They explained that her immune system wasn't strong enough yet, so we shouldn't let anyone get too close. We had that warning in mind as we made our way out of the hospital. It was easy enough to avoid people in the hallways, but when we arrived in the lobby, it was packed. We couldn't believe it. Everywhere we looked, it was wall-to-wall people.

It turned out that they were filming a scene from the now iconic TV series *Dallas* starring Larry Hagman, Linda Gray, and Victoria Principal. It seemed like almost everyone was a fan of the show at the time. We were pretty nervous as we made our way through such a big crowd, but fortunately, everyone was so focused on the spectacle of the TV production that no one even noticed the new baby. We made it through without having to stop even once. Then, at long last, we got to take Ashley home.

Chapter 5

ADJUSTMENT

AFTER ASHLEY WAS BORN, our main focus was getting her to a place where she would be strong enough to come home from the hospital. Of course, once that happened, our difficulties weren't over. I was home with a newborn who wasn't entirely out of the woods yet, and for all intents and purposes, I was legally blind.

The issues with my eyes—and the laser surgeries I had to stanch the bleeding—would continue for years. Eventually I would get my sight back, but first I had to figure out how to manage it all and manage being a new mother at the same time. Before we left the NICU, I didn't have a real sense of how tough that would be. When things were starting to look up for Ashley, I remember saying to one of the nurses at the hospital, "I'll sure be glad when this is all over and we can go home. When that happens, I'm going to come back and volunteer here because I'm so grateful for everything you've done for us."

The nurse didn't say anything, but she gave me a look like I was out of my mind. Looking back now, it is pretty funny that I thought I would have time to volunteer with all that was going on in my life.

In the beginning, David picked up a lot of the caretaking duties that were more difficult for me because of my sight issues. I was advised not to breastfeed because of the medications I was on for diabetes, so we had to give Ashley formula, which meant that he could feed her without me. He was the one who got up in the middle of the night when Ashley needed to be fed or soothed.

Of course, David had to work during the day, and he traveled frequently, so my mother came for a while. Eventually, though, she had to get back home, so bright woman that she is, she came up with the idea of getting a college student, someone from the same sorority that I had once pledged, to come and help me out. She contacted Southern Methodist University, near where we lived in Dallas, to see if they could arrange something.

We really lucked out because the young woman who answered our call just loved babies. I thought we would end up with someone who simply needed a part-time job, which would have been fine, but this young woman was clearly well off, always going to expensive restaurants with her friends and having her own car to drive. It didn't seem like she needed the money. She was just happy to help. She spent a year with us, driving me to doctor's appointments and on errands, looking after little Ashley when I had my eye treatments. She became like a part of the family for a little while.

Thanks to all the help we were lucky enough to receive, as well as some flexibility and patience on our part, we were able to muddle through. It helped that Ashley was a really good baby. Just like when I was pregnant, my eyesight would ebb and flow. About four months after she was born, I was finally able to see well enough to distinguish the freckles on Ashley's nose. It was a momentous occasion for me. I looked at them and said, "I knew those were there!" In my mind, when I imagined what my daughter looked like, I always pictured her with freckles on her face. And I had been right!

LIFE HAS A WAY OF CHUGGING ALONG no matter what you're going through, and that's how it was for us. There was nothing to do but adapt and keep up.

I credit my parents, particularly my dad, for instilling that attitude in me. Whenever I had a setback, I was bound and determined not to let it stand in my way. I couldn't ignore what my body was going through entirely—"You have to follow the rules of diabetes," as Dad would always say—but it didn't stop me from getting on with my life and getting the most out of it that I could.

The effect the pregnancy had on me physically was the first big setback I'd experienced in my life as a result of having diabetes. But look what I got out of it in the process! An amazing daughter whom I have been grateful for every day since.

Of course, it wasn't the last setback I would have. The next came not long after. When I first decided I wanted to try to get pregnant, my endocrinologist had been optimistic about my prospects, in large part because my diabetes had been fairly stable up until that point in my life. But after what I went through to have Ashley, the calculus changed. In fact, my obstetrician/gynecologist (OB/GYN) was adamant in his opinion: he didn't think that I should ever get pregnant again.

Based on his recommendation, I scheduled a tubal ligation (more commonly known as "having your tubes tied") to make sure that I didn't. I already had an eye surgery scheduled, so it was decided that both procedures could be done at once while I was already under anesthesia.

Just before the surgery, I talked to my OB/GYN again and told him that I wasn't entirely certain that I didn't want more children. It hadn't been easy, of course, but I had made it through pregnancy once, and I was still holding out hope that I could do it again. But he was having none of it. He got up real close, just inches from my face, when he said to me: "If you put your body through that kind of stress, you will become permanently blind and who knows what else. You won't be able to live a normal life. You can never do this again."

I think I needed to hear it told to me that starkly in order to believe it. I'd always been good at pushing past the potential limitations of my diabetes, but there is such a thing as taking it too far. My doctor was letting me know where that line was and warning me, in no uncertain terms, not to cross it.

So I went ahead with the surgery. I wanted to be there for Ashley and David for years to come, and I figured that this was what I needed to do to ensure that would happen.

Diabetic Retinopathy

Diabetic retinopathy is a complication of diabetes where the vessels in the retina, at the back of the eye, become damaged. They can swell up and leak, or they can become blocked, which can cause abnormal new blood vessels to grow to compensate for the lack of blood supply.

Pregnancy can put someone with diabetes at higher risk, but anyone with any type of diabetes can develop retinopathy. Proper management of blood sugar levels along with blood pressure and cholesterol levels (which can also put a person at higher risk if not managed properly) is the best way to guard against it as well as being on the lookout for symptoms, which can include the following:

- Changes in vision, which may come and go

- Blurred vision or vision loss

- Seeing spots, streaks, or floaters

AS I ALREADY WROTE, I always had this sense that I would see again, so I never felt panicked about my sight loss. It was more a frustration than anything else, but I understood that it was going to take time. And it certainly did. Ashley was four years old, and we had moved on to Wichita, Kansas, by the time I had another vitrectomy for my eyes. David had gotten a new job running marketing at Pizza Hut by then, so that had necessitated the move.

When I went for the operation, David came with me, as did a pile of his work, which he was busily looking through as I was being prepped for surgery. It wasn't his fault. I'd been through so many eye procedures by that point that this just felt like another day at the hospital for him. I had to remind him that this was a real operation this time and a much bigger deal than before. Rather than just lasering dry the bleeding vessels, they were going in to surgically remove the damaged tissue, which would improve my vision and alleviate the need for regular procedures. It didn't take much for him to get the hint and put the work away.

I did get my sight back, though not entirely. It would never again be as sharp as it once had been. I tried to continue playing tennis for a while, but I couldn't see the ball as well as I used to. I was able to drive again, but I felt like I had to be a lot more careful. I would drive slowly and get honked at all the time. After that I felt a bit guilty about all the times I'd gotten frustrated with someone on the road. I thought to myself, *I'm never going to honk at a slow person again because they're just doing the best they can!*

The relative stability I'd always had never fully returned either. I started to have more episodes where I'd need an additional shot of insulin if my blood sugar was too high or, as more often happened, where I would suffer lows and needed sugar to stabilize. That usually came in the form of Pepsi for me because it was what I found generally worked the best.

Unlike when I was growing up, diabetes wasn't a totally hidden or taboo subject in our house. I didn't talk about it a lot outside the family, but Ashley grew up knowing about it, knowing what to do if I had an episode, and even how to give me shots. When she was only about six or seven, I got up one morning to make her breakfast. My blood sugar was so low that I ended up wilting to the floor. I didn't quite faint, but I wasn't all there either. Ashley found me and knew what to do. Without any prompting, she went straight to the fridge, got me a Pepsi, opened it herself, and helped me drink some.

After I started feeling a little better, I said to her, "Thank you, honey. I really appreciate you for helping."

She just looked at me and said, "Well, Mom, I need to eat." She wanted breakfast, and she understood what she needed to do to get it. She was so young that she doesn't even remember that episode, but I sure do.

In fact, Ashley remembers being more concerned at that age about me drinking too much coffee than about the fact that I had diabetes. She'd learned in school about the effects of caffeine, so that seemed like the bigger deal, more sinister than the shots she saw me take every day.

I hardly remember any such incidents with my father. My younger sister, Cindy, doesn't either, although she's sure that he must have had them. (We always had orange juice in the house, which may have been because it's often used like I use Pepsi, to quickly get sugar into someone and bring them out of a low.) We just weren't aware of them. Two of Cindy's three children have type 1 diabetes, and she believes that both of us would be able to spot Dad having a low in a heartbeat now, with all that we've experienced over the years, but back then, because we never talked about it, we never learned what to look for with Dad like Ashley did with me.

That doesn't mean it was always easy for Ashley. She remembers one time when she was in seventh grade and her dad was out of town. I had such an extreme low that she couldn't get me to drink any of the Pepsi she was trying to coax into me. Usually she could get through to me when I was in a state like that. I always heard her through whatever fog I was in and would do what she asked because I always wanted to get back to her. But this time, I was completely unresponsive, so she had to call 911 and go with me in an ambulance to the hospital.

I never wanted my diabetes to impact Ashley, but I guess it was inevitable that it would. It's one of the hardest things to accept as a parent, I think: the fact that all of us—all the good parts as well as all our struggles—impact our kids. But she has turned out to be such a wonderful woman with three beautiful children of her own that it's hard to harbor too many regrets. Diabetes is simply a fact of life for me, and yet I still really wanted to be her mom. And as Ashley now puts it, "I always knew how much I was wanted because I knew Mom went through hell to get me."

BECOMING A MOM AND EXPERIENCING changes in my health weren't the only things I had to adjust to during those years. At the same time, David's career was taking off. When we left Dallas, where Ashley was born, and moved to Wichita, David had taken a job as the head of marketing at Pizza Hut, which was part of the PepsiCo system. That was the beginning of a new phase in his career, and he kept climbing the corporate ladder from there.

PepsiCo had divisions all over the country at the time. Its corporate headquarters was in Purchase, New York, and the Pepsi-Cola Company was in Somers, New York. It also owned several brands, including Taco Bell, which was based in Irvine, California; Frito-Lay, which was in Dallas; Pizza Hut, which was in Wichita, Kansas; and KFC, which was in Louisville, Kentucky. I told David that I supported his career, and I understood that he needed to follow the opportunities where they led him, but the only place where I really, really didn't want to end up was Louisville. That was where I'd spent my high school years, and I'd intentionally made the decision to leave it behind when I chose to go to college in Missouri. I'd done that because I wanted a new experience in a new place, and I didn't want to go backward.

After he cut his teeth working as the head of marketing at Pizza Hut in Wichita for four years, David got a job as executive vice president of marketing and sales at the Pepsi-Cola Company, which meant a move to Connecticut. The housing market there was much more expensive than it was in Wichita, so I was skeptical when David said he found the perfect house for us in the town of Wilton. Built in 1930, it had once been owned by Johnny Gruelle, an author and illustrator who is best known as the creator of the children's characters Raggedy Ann and Andy. It was situated next to a river, and the property was dotted with apple trees. There was a fireplace in one of the bedrooms with original tile that Gruelle had decorated with Raggedy Ann and Andy figures. It even had a ballroom (not that we planned to throw any balls) and had been written up in the *New York Times* because it was so charming.

I didn't even want to see it because I thought it sounded too good to be true and that we wouldn't be able to afford it, but David insisted. In the end, we were able to get an incredible deal on it because the previous owners had started construction but never finished. Still, I wasn't convinced. We were getting a deal, but it wasn't exactly cheap, and I became aware of the fact that the previous six people who had occupied David's new position had been fired by the company. I said I would only agree to buy the house if PepsiCo gave David a letter promising they would buy it from us if David became "terminated employee number seven." To both our surprise, they agreed, and we moved into the house.

I loved living in Connecticut. We were close enough to New York City that we'd go into the city about once a month to see a Broadway play. We'd drive around during the fall months to see the leaves change colors. It was magnificent and a far cry from the scarcity of trees we had in the prairielands of Kansas. I also decided during that time to go back to school and get my master's degree in social work at Columbia University. As part of the program, I worked with kids who had diabetes. I remember leading a class once where I had all the kids draw a picture of what they thought their diabetes looked like. I did it too, and colored mine like there was a fire burning inside my body. My professors questioned whether that was the right approach—to show an image that could be perceived as negative by the kids—but I felt it was honest. Diabetes felt to me like this fire inside that I constantly needed to tamp down or even quell if it started to get too big or out of control. I thought that kids with diabetes would relate to that. I still think that many of them did.

It was while I was earning my degree that I was finally able to deal with something I'd been struggling with for years: an eating disorder. I learned that eating disorders are fairly common among people with diabetes (both types, but especially type 1), which isn't all that surprising when I started to think more about it. My struggles with food began when I was quite young and battled with my mother over what she made me eat. The lack of choices and control was difficult for me, and I learned pretty early how to adopt some secretive behaviors around what I was eating. My eating disorder—which took the form of bulimia—didn't start until I was in my twenties, but I think the groundwork was laid well before that.

When it started, David and I were living in Pittsburgh and working together at the ad agency. It's hard to say exactly why something like this happens, but I have learned that many people with diabetes struggle with issues around self-esteem, and I know I wasn't entirely happy with how things were going in my life at the time. We got married so young, and we had previously lived near his family in Maryland. For the first time, it was just the two of us, entirely on our own. Working together at the same place on top of that probably wasn't the best situation. I often compared myself to David even though we were in different departments, and it always felt like he was thriving while I was just doing OK. The truth was that he didn't feel like he was thriving then either, but that's not how I saw things at the time.

I had been able to curb my eating disorder, like I did my drinking, while I was pregnant with Ashley. It was important to me to do that for her, but after she was born, I picked the habit back up again. In addition to helping control my weight after gaining so much during the pregnancy, the behavior also helped me control my blood sugar spikes. I often simply wasn't consuming enough food to raise my sugar levels. Of course, I started having a lot more lows as a result. Eating disorders come with a greater chance of serious complications when you have diabetes because of how important it is to maintain a stable blood sugar while continuing to provide healthy fuel for the body, so it was obviously a very disruptive pattern.

And it was a pattern I had a devil of a time getting over. It's one of the reasons why I chose to pursue a degree in social work. It gave me a chance to learn more about human behavior, including my own. During that period, I worked one-on-one with a counselor who taught me how to use behavioral therapy techniques to change what had become some long-standing habits by then. It wasn't easy, but with time and persistence, it worked for me. I started to feel a greater sense of control over my food choices and my life in general.

For many years my bulimia was one of those things, like diabetes, that I felt like I shouldn't talk about, but I'm gradually learning to see my ability to bounce back from setbacks as one of my biggest strengths. It turns out that there's always more to learn in life, and in talking with family members and friends as I wrote this book, I found that people continually remarked on that particular kind of strength I have. They called me things like "brave," "resilient," "remarkable," "a fighter," even "an inspiration."

I have to admit that it's hard for me to even write these things because those are words I would never use to describe myself. But it's also quite something to get a chance to see yourself through other peoples' eyes. I feel grateful to be seen that way, and it makes me wonder if I was right all those years ago, as a social work student, when I wanted to draw that fire inside me despite the hesitancy of my professors. Now I wonder if it wasn't my diabetes that I was picturing after all but the real essence of who I am. I think it may be that fire inside me that kept me going through whatever challenges I've faced. It's that fire inside me that has always spurred me to get back up no matter how hard I've been knocked down. And perhaps that fire inside me is a quality that's well worth talking about, even something (dare I say it?) to be proud of.

ALL IN ALL, LIFE IN CONNECTICUT was pretty good for us. All three of us thought so, but after only four years there, David came home with what he thought was exciting news. By then, he had set his sights on running one of the PepsiCo divisions one day—it was the big goal he had set for himself—and he was finally getting the chance. So he was brimming with excitement when he said to Ashley, "Guess what? Your dad is going to be president!"

She thought he meant president of Pepsi, so she was excited for him at first, but when he clarified that he had been offered the job of president of KFC, which meant a move to Louisville, she burst into tears. She would have to leave her home and all her friends behind. She was in the middle of the school year at the time, as was I. Columbia was just a short train ride away from where we lived in Wilton, and I was still finishing up my degree.

It was too big of an opportunity to pass up, of course, so David took the job in Louisville while Ashley and I stayed behind to finish out the school year. That meant several months apart while David commuted back and forth between Connecticut and Kentucky. It's funny now to think about how reluctant we were about the move at first, because all of us, including Ashley (who is now grown with her own family) have made a life in Louisville and feel so tied to the community. But at the time, it felt like another adjustment we had to figure out how to make work for all of us.

Chapter 6

ACCEPTANCE

EVEN THOUGH I CONTINUED to have issues with my eyesight and my diabetes would never again be as stable as it had been before my pregnancy, I never wanted to be the kind of person who felt like I couldn't do things because of my condition. As a child, the notion was instilled in me early that I always had a choice about how I handled my diabetes. My choice, more often than not, has been to accept my condition as something I need to monitor but that doesn't have to get in the way of prioritizing the things in life that give me joy, even when it's hard sometimes. For me, that means focusing on things like family, community, traveling to new places, learning new things, and entertaining the people who are important in my life.

It's a good thing, too, that those were my personal priorities, because they dovetailed well with what was happening in David's career. When he set his sights on "running something someday,"

I don't think even he knew how far that aspiration would take him. I sure didn't. Our life in Louisville became more and more entrenched as he rose through the company ranks to eventually become the CEO of Yum! Brands, a Fortune 500 company with one and a half million employees around the world that encompasses the well-known restaurant brands of KFC, Taco Bell, and Pizza Hut. As that was happening, things like traveling and entertaining became regular parts of our life together.

One prime example is the festivities we took part in every year surrounding one of the city's most defining events: the Kentucky Derby. Even though I spent the latter part of my childhood in Louisville, I'd never paid a whole lot of attention to the Derby growing up. I remember watching it on TV with my family but never much more than that. In fact, when I was in high school, I worked at a dress shop on Saturdays when the Derby was taking place, so I often missed it entirely. Years later, when Yum! Brands became the first sponsor of the event, David and I got to watch the race from box seats on the finish line. I used to sit there in wonder thinking about how completely life can change and how it can take you places you never even thought to dream of before.

The Derby is always held on the first Saturday in May, but the build-up begins weeks in advance. Around town you will hear people talking about all the different jockeys and which horses are favored to win. People start planning their outfits well in advance because the Derby is definitely a dress-up occasion. "Dressier than church clothes," I would often counsel guests coming in from out of town when they asked about it. And if you want to be with it, you need to wear a hat, often one large and elaborately adorned in bright spring colors like pink, yellow, and red.

Because David's company was hosting, we'd often have around eighty people coming into town for the event, and we would host them for more than just the main race. While the Derby race itself is well known for being the most famous ninety seconds in sports, the pomp and circumstance surrounding it goes on for days. We'd plan outings leading up to the main event, like rounds of golf or a trip to the breeding farms in nearby Lexington. It may sound like an odd thing to some, but watching the horses breed is something of a tradition. Of course, if you've seen a horse breed once, you've seen it a thousand times—at least that's how I looked at it—so I had more fun watching people's reaction to the spectacle. After doing that a few times, I started to notice a pattern. When the "event" commenced, the women would generally lean in to get a closer look, while the men would take a step back and cross their arms. I don't know what that says about the difference between the genders, but I couldn't help but enjoy seeing the same reactions repeat themselves year after year after year.

Placing your bets is as much a part of the experience as wearing a hat, even if it's only a small token bet. Our first year I won almost $2,000 by picking the winner of both the Kentucky Oaks and the Kentucky Derby. The Oaks is a shorter race of only fillies (female horses) that takes place on Friday, the day before the Derby. My friend Molly Neher, who came twice with her husband, Tim, won one year after she picked a horse based solely on its name, which was similar to the name of someone she knew.

My reasons for choosing a particular horse were about as scientific as Molly's, but I won big that first year all the same, and I was hooked after that. Sadly, even though I continued to bet year after year for more than a decade, I never won again.

Then there's the food. One friend described it as eating for three days straight. We hosted a lot of brunches that flowed into lunches that flowed into cocktail hours and hors d'oeuvres that were followed by formal dinners. Sometimes we'd put up tents in the backyard to host events at our home. Other times, we'd rent out places like the Louisville Art Museum or Locust Grove, which is a historic home in town. The traditional mint julep was always on offer as were a lot of Southern staples like cheese grits and country ham. Generally speaking, it was not great food for someone with diabetes, especially the juleps, which contained both bourbon and a good bit of sugar, but you can bet I would have some anyway. I always had to join in the fun.

Even just getting to Churchill Downs, the track where the race takes place, was a production. Our whole group of eighty or so people would travel together in a caravan of limousines from whichever venue we'd chosen that year to host the prerace brunch. The local police would stop traffic on the expressway so we could pass, with police cars stationed at each exit to block them off and motorcycled policemen racing ahead to clear the way. It would take something like thirty limos to transport everyone, and the company had to rent them from as far away as Kansas City and Wichita because there were never enough available in the rather modest-sized city of Louisville. Our neighbors would sometimes give us a hard time about it all, especially when brunch was held at our house and the parade of limos left from there. "Some people will do anything for attention," they'd say, but it was all in good fun, and truthfully it was that caravan that many of our guests liked the best and remember the most.

The Kentucky Derby is often called the most popular horse race in the world, and it's watched by millions of people. An event like that naturally attracts celebrities, and since we're lucky enough to have three guest rooms, some of them even stayed at our house. One memorable guest was professional golfer Arnold Palmer, who came with his wife, Kit. One morning, I was up early having my coffee in the kitchen when Arnold walked in. We'd been chatting for a bit when I accidentally knocked over a glass. Without missing a beat, he said to me, "Where's your broom?" I protested, of course, because I couldn't have any guest, let alone this famous man, cleaning up after me in my own home. But he insisted. "Oh honey," he said, "I've been cleaning up ever since I was a boy in Latrobe, Pennsylvania." He was so charming about it that I gave in. Then I stood and watched as he got down on his hands and knees on my kitchen floor and cleared up the whole mess for me. I know he was this legendary athlete and everything, but that moment is what really impressed me about him. Later that weekend he gave me a pair of beautiful blue earrings as a thank-you gift for hosting him and his wife. He said he'd chosen them because they matched my eyes. He really was quite a charmer. David likes to joke that he's amazed he still had a chance with me after all that.

Singer-songwriter Brad Paisley came one year, too, and because my birthday is in early May and often coincides with Derby festivities, David convinced him to surprise me by singing "Happy Birthday" after dinner that night, which he did while using a beer bottle in place of a pick to play the tune on his guitar. Actress Fran Drescher came one year, too, as did the Blues Brothers, the comedy team of Dan Aykroyd and John Belushi from *Saturday Night Live*. The Blues Brothers didn't stay with us but instead came by to get ready before one of the events, so I offered them our guest suite in the basement. When I did that, I'd forgotten that the shower down there was only stocked with dog shampoo because that's where we always washed our golden retriever. I didn't realize my mistake until after they left, so I never got a chance to apologize. I had to hope they didn't take offense. In any case, they never mentioned it, so hopefully they didn't notice, and the doggie shampoo did the trick!

I always loved the ritual of it all, but I admit it could be pretty stressful too. By the time Sunday evening rolled around and everyone had gone home, David and I would be ready to crawl into bed. It was always important to me that everybody have a good time, and I took pride and pleasure in being the hostess and first lady of Yum! Brands, but sometimes playing that role and being on all the time took a toll. One year I went into diabetic shock when we were still at Churchill Downs. I passed out when we were leaving the track, and David took me in his arms and carried me to an ambulance. (He kids me that in my fancy dress, it was like having Cinderella in his arms, only I had on both my

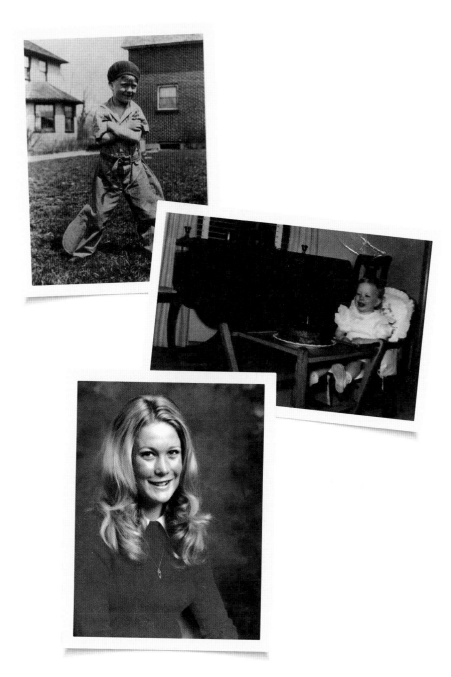

1   Jack Henderson, my father, was diagnosed with type 1 diabetes at the age of four. Isn't he cute? (1930)

2   My cute first birthday photo! (1953)

3   My classic senior year photo from my time at Atherton High School in Louisville, Kentucky. (1970)

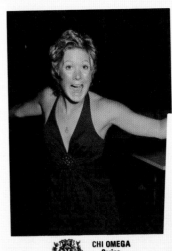

CHI OMEGA
Casino
March 23, 1974

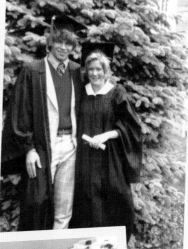

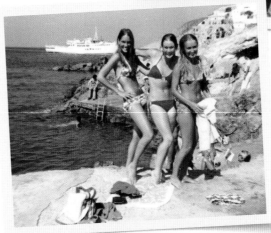

1   I clearly enjoyed the freedom of college and always love a good party. (1974)

2   We made it! David and I both graduated from the School of Journalism at the University of Missouri in May of 1974.

3   Me and my college girlfriends in Capri, Greece, without a care in the world in the summer of 1974.

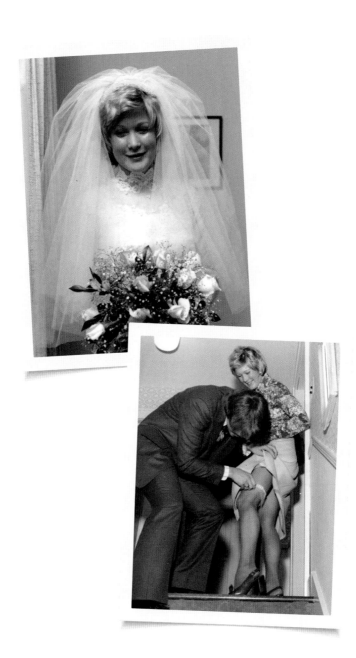

1   I married David Novak on a
    cold, rainy day in Louisville,
    Kentucky, in 1974. I still believe
    rainy days are lucky days.

2   David and I just got married . . .
    Oh, boy, here comes the
    honeymoon!

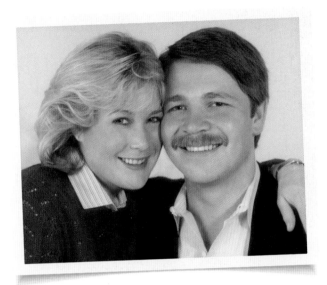

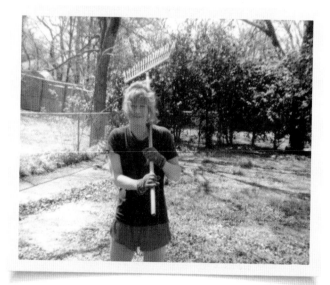

1   Our first formal portrait as a married couple. David thought his mustache made him look older. (1975)

2   I love working with my hands, including raking leaves at our first house in Dallas, Texas. (1979)

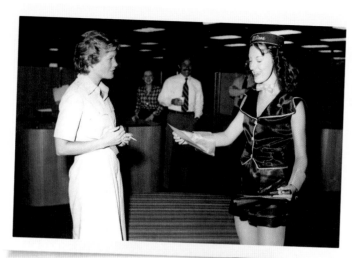

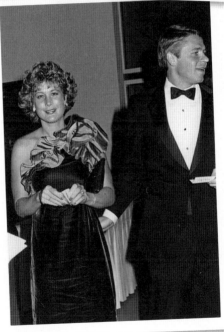

1   My favorite job was in television sales for WFAA, where I was recognized as salesperson of the year in 1980.

2   David and I dressed to impress for a formal affair in Dallas, Texas. (1980)

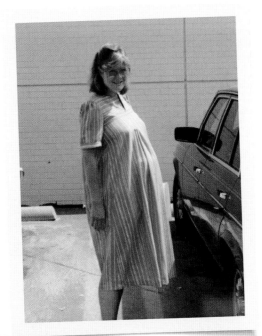

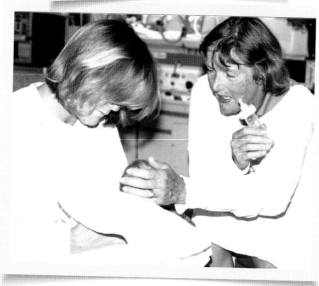

1   Weighing in at 172 pounds waiting
    for my four-pound, ten-ounce baby.
    (1983)

2   My mom, Ann, was delighted with
    the arrival of Ashley in June of 1983.
    She always thought I could have
    children despite the warnings.

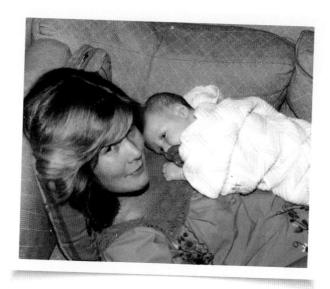

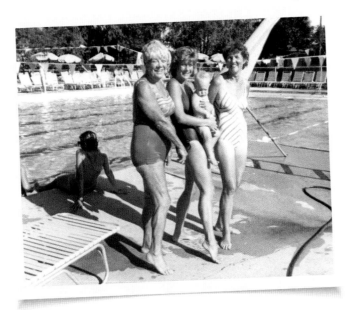

1   I loved cuddle time and 4:00 p.m. naps
    with my daughter, Ashley. (1983)

2   All Henderson women are great swimmers.
    Here we are showing our personality
    by the pool in 1984! Left to right: my
    grandmother, Helen Bjorklund; me with
    Ashley; and my mom, Ann Henderson.

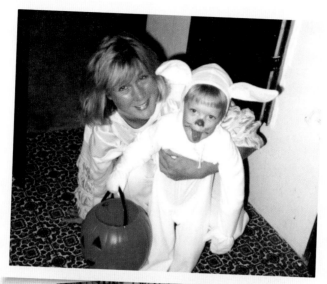

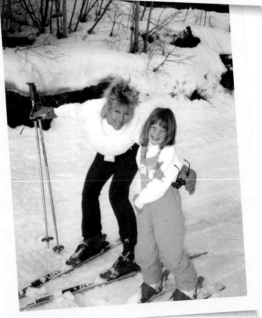

1   I love celebrating every holiday, including Halloween 1985 with my bunny child, Ashley.

2   The only time that Ashley and I were standing up that entire day in Steamboat Springs! (1988)

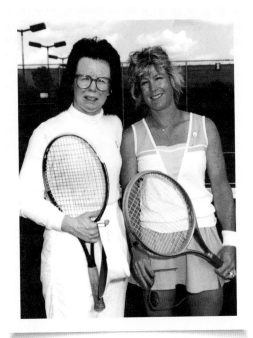

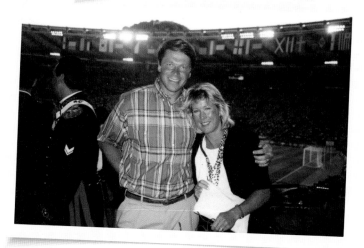

1   My one-on-one with Billie Jean King . . .
     She won. (1988)

2   I am always up for a good time with David,
     and I love attending sporting events,
     including the 1990 World Cup in Italy.

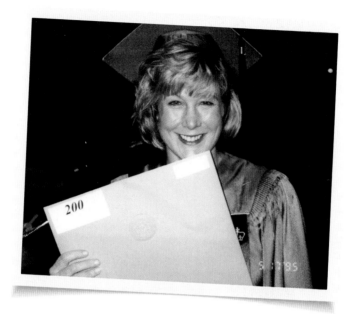

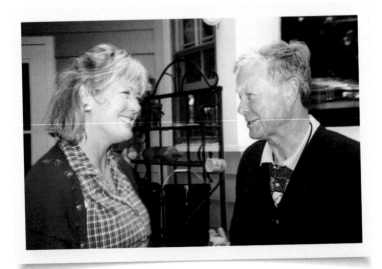

1   I worked hard and earned my master of social work degree from Columbia University in New York City in 1995.

2   Dad and I had a very special relationship. He always knew just what to say to put a smile on my face. (1998)

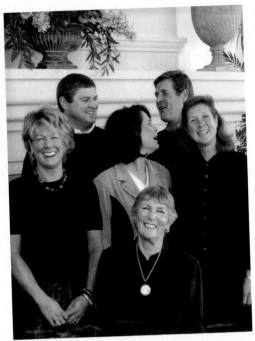

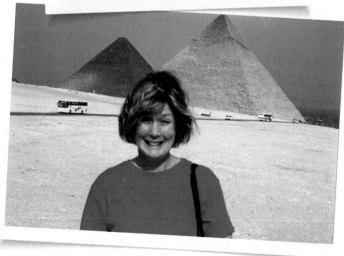

1   My siblings and I could never all look at
    the camera at the same time. Left to right:
    me, Rick, Cindy, Ann, Jeff, and Gretchen.
    (2000)

2   I got to travel the world, weathering the wind
    at the pyramids. (2000)

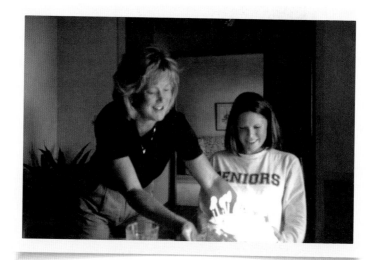

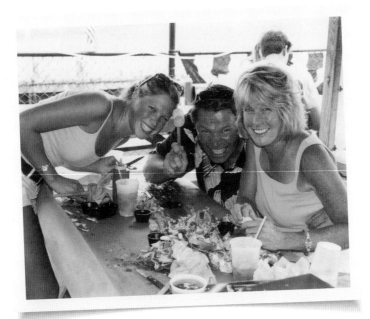

1   Every year is a gift and should be
    celebrated to the fullest. (2002)

2   David, Ashley, and I love to explore
    new cities and especially the new food.
    (2000)

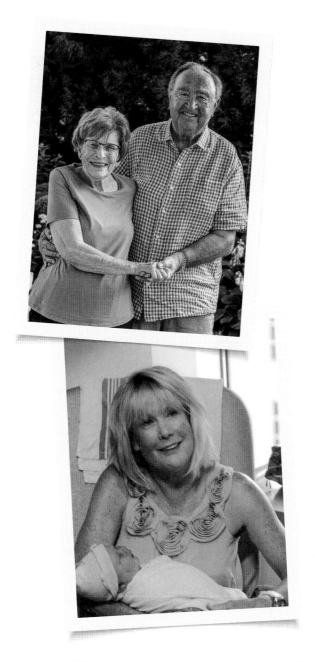

1 I married into the wild Novak family, and Jean and Charles Novak loved me like their own. (2019)

2 Audrey Louise is my first grandchild, and she was named in my honor. (2010)

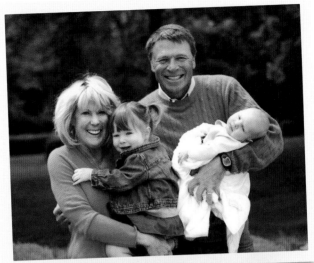

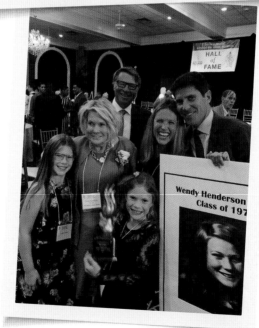

1   My grandchildren call me "Gigi," which stands for "Gorgeous Grandma," and David "Ogo," which stands for "Oh, Great One." Why not make up your own grandparent name?

2   I was inducted into the Atherton High School Hall of Fame, finally earning some bling. Left to right: Audrey, me, David, Claire, Ashley, and Jonathan. (2019)

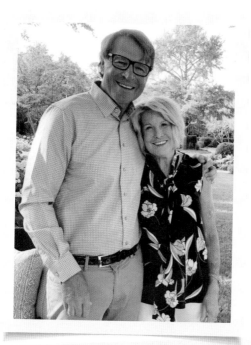

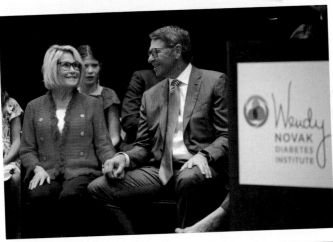

1   David and I enjoying retired life. No haircuts required once you're retired. (2020)

2   A wonderful day watching Ashley announce the $15 million gift to Norton Healthcare that created the Wendy Novak Diabetes Institute. (2022)

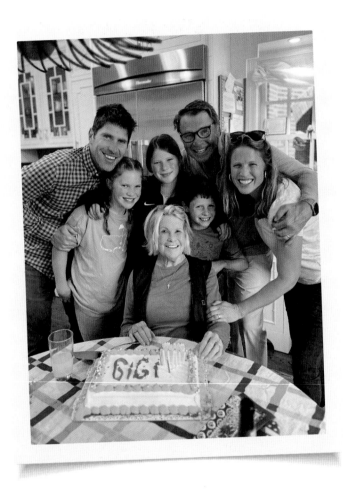

My family celebrating my seventy-first birthday in our typical fashion!
Left to right: Jonathan, Claire, Audrey, Luke, David, and Ashley. (2023)

shoes.) At the time, there were 150,000 people streaming out of the track, so it was no easy feat getting to the hospital. Once we made it, however, the doctors were able to bring me back into balance—they always do. My biggest concern at the time was that our houseguests had to have dinner by themselves.

Too much stress is hard on anyone's health, but it can be particularly complicated when you have diabetes. The hormones the body releases when it's under stress can cause your blood sugar to rise. For me, however, stress often has the opposite effect of bottoming out my blood sugar. That's probably because stressful times pull my focus away from what I need to do to remain stable. I'll be busy running around and forget to eat. I might not be as diligent about monitoring my blood sugar levels and taking my medication. A ready supply of alcohol at parties and events like the Derby certainly doesn't help. Drinking alcohol can contribute to lows too, especially for people with type 1 diabetes. It didn't help that endocrinologists were in short supply in the area at that time. When we first moved to Louisville, it took four months to get an appointment with one.

None of that stopped me, however, from doing it all over again year after year. Not just the Derby, either, but a whole lot more. We hosted a Christmas party every year at our home for Yum! employees, which started a tradition of doing the house up each year with rather elaborate holiday decorations. That was in addition to all the other events I attended, out-of-town business associates I hosted, and the traveling I did to support David in his role as CEO. At least one weekend a month was dedicated to one of these things, and sometimes more. I suppose I could have pulled back and taken on fewer responsibilities, but that wasn't what I wanted. Sure, it could be stressful, and if I'm completely honest, sometimes it got to be too much. I ended up in the hospital more than once. But at the same time, I always knew how lucky I was to lead the life I was leading, and I was determined to make the most of it.

Stress and Diabetes

Stress is the body's natural reaction to difficult or threatening events or circumstances, and it's something that we all experience from time to time. Of course, we also know that too much of it can negatively impact our health. That's particularly true for people with diabetes. Emotional, psychological, and physical stress can impact them in the following ways:

- When stressed, their bodies make certain hormones that can raise blood sugar.

- Stress can serve as a distraction, causing people to forget to take medications or focus less on managing their blood sugar.

- Stress is often associated with changes in behavior that can affect a person's ability to manage their diabetes, like changes in diet, schedule, and activity levels or exercise, which can result in either high or low blood sugar, depending on the behavior.

Our first year at the Derby, the local newspaper took a picture of me in my bright pink St. John outfit with my matching pink hat. In the photo, I'm looking up at David after he just said something that totally melted me. He'd been telling me how much he loved our life together in Kentucky and how lucky he felt to be able to enjoy moments like this one. I felt exactly the same way. In fact, in that moment, I thought David Novak hung the moon, and you can see it written all over my face. I still feel that way about him. Through all our ups and downs, it's hard to imagine wanting our life to be any different.

BACK WHEN I WAS FINDING WAYS to pass the time while confined to the family sick room as a kid, I never imagined, even as I was looking at all those travel posters my mom posted on the walls, that I would one day get to travel the world. But Yum! Brands is an international company, so I've since gotten a chance to see every one of the places pictured in those posters plus so many more.

We've been to Egypt where, in the little rustic town in the shadow of the great pyramids at Giza, there's a combination KFC and Pizza Hut. David calls it his "proudest and most embarrassing moment as CEO" because while it's really something to see how far the company's reach has extended, it also felt like the restaurant's red roof and neon sign stuck out in the little desert town. It was like the restaurant was intruding on the majestic history of the place.

When we arrived in the country, one of the first things I noticed were all the armed guards on the streets and in front of our hotel. One day I wanted to go to the shops to see if I could find an amulet necklace, a kind of good luck charm that I'd seen people wearing. As I tried to leave the hotel, a man who worked there stopped me and told me, in broken English, that I couldn't go. I didn't understand him at first, but it turned out that he was trying to tell me that it was too dangerous to go out on my own. I wasn't looking for trouble, of course, but I also didn't like the idea of being told I couldn't do something, so I arranged to go another time with a guide to find the souvenir I was looking for.

We got to go on safari in South Africa one year as well after visiting KFC locations in Johannesburg and Cape Town. Ashley was grown by then and married to her husband, Jon, so they came along with us. We saw all of what are known as "the big five" animals—elephants, leopards, lions, rhinoceroses, and cape buffalo—which are what big game hunters once named the five beasts they considered to be the hardest and most dangerous to hunt. We weren't hunting, of course, just hoping to catch a glimpse of them, which we did and then some. We saw impalas running all over the place, baboons who liked to break into camp and steal beer and Snickers bars out of the fridge, whole prides of lions eating their latest catch (I couldn't help but note that the mothers in the pride always ate last), two rhinos fighting each other, and even an elephant that charged the jeep we were riding in. That scared even our guides, and the driver managed to steer us out of the way just in time.

For me, almost as impressive as all the wildlife were the stars in the sky at night. I hadn't been able to see stars well in years because of my waning eyesight, but they were so bright and so numerous there that I could see them quite clearly. I'll never forget feeling like I could reach up and grab a whole handful of them. It was really something to be able to experience seeing them again after so long. I was also proud of myself by the end for never having a diabetes-related incident during the entire two weeks we were away. I suppose I was able to do what was necessary to survive in the wild!

Yum! Brands also had a big presence in China, so we have visited the country numerous times over the years. I still have vivid memories of taking a special trip with a group from the company to see the life-size terracotta warriors in Xi'an, about an hour and a half outside Beijing. The sculptures—which number in the thousands, stand as high as six feet tall, and are accompanied by terracotta horses and chariots—were created in the third century to guard the tomb of Qin Shi Huang, the first emperor of a unified China. What struck me most about them is the fact that each of their faces appears to be unique, with different shapes, details, and expressions. That, and the fact that they were buried there for more than 1,700 years before some local farmers discovered them in 1974, completely by accident, as they set out to dig a new well.

We went to the Beijing Summer Olympics in 2008, where we got to see both the diving and the swimming competitions. I'd been a lifeguard and competitive swimmer in junior high and high school, so those events were particularly fun to see. However, when we arrived in Beijing that year, it was about 105 degrees and humid, not exactly hospitable weather, and David had plans for us to play golf with some of his colleagues. I loved swimming, and I used to be a pretty good tennis player before my eyesight started to fade, but unlike David, I've never been very good at golf. Still, I was determined not to be left behind. I wouldn't give up even though, as David lovingly put it, I "set an all-time record for number of strokes played in a round of golf."

By the time we reached the sixteenth hole, everyone was drenched in sweat. "You know, Wendy, we could just call it quits," they said to me after I'd hit the ball so many times that everyone had lost count. But I was bound and determined to finish no matter how long it took. I guess that might seem a little prideful, but David is always quick to point out that that quality of mine is also a strength. I am a determined person. I believe in persevering, no matter what. Sometimes when I encounter challenges, particularly with my health, all I have is my belief that I can get through it and get back on my feet again. Perhaps that's why I was so taken with those terracotta warriors who, for more than a thousand years, endured in that field even after they'd been buried and forgotten. They are a monument to real endurance.

That's the thing about endurance: you never really know how much of it you have until it's tested. My belief that I could last the distance allowed me to go to some amazing places and do some amazing things. I never wanted to be the kind of person who stayed home and worried about whether or not I could take it, and so I didn't.

IT WAS IMPORTANT TO ME to keep living my life, but traveling wasn't always easy. For my friend Jenny Cottingham's fiftieth birthday, I went with a group of girlfriends to Mexico. Our last night there, we were out quite late celebrating. On the way back to where we were staying, some in our group wanted to stop for food, so I stayed in the car with Jenny and my friend Barbie Sweet while the others went inside. We'd had quite a bit to drink, plus we'd been going and going all day long. It was all probably a bit too much for me. It must have been, because I passed out in the car, and my friends couldn't wake me up.

This is middle-of-nowhere Mexico, mind you, so none of my friends had any idea where to go to get help. Jenny called her sister in Chicago, who is a doctor, and she said they needed to get me to an emergency room right away. I don't remember any of what happened next, but my friends tell me that we were lucky to have a really nice taxi driver. It was late at night—or, more accurately, really early in the morning—but he knew of somewhere that was open at that hour. It wasn't a hospital exactly, more like an urgent care place. It was tiny and somewhat run-down, but there was a doctor there who, even though his English was limited and my friends' Spanish was nonexistent, managed to figure out what I needed with the help of Jenny's sister, who was doing her best to translate through the phone.

The next thing I remember is waking up to the sound of a rooster crowing somewhere nearby. Thankfully, a couple of my friends had stayed with me through the night, because I had no idea where I was. I had been out for several hours, but I was well enough by then to not only leave the clinic but also fly home later that same day.

Traveling can be challenging for people with diabetes. Your regular schedule gets disrupted. You may be more active than usual, and you may end up eating differently than you usually do. There may be a time change, which can mess up your medication schedule. For my sixtieth birthday, a group of girlfriends went with me to Hong Kong (which is twelve hours ahead of Louisville), and I ended up in the hospital there as well.

Once again, we were celebrating, so of course I wanted to see everything I could possibly see and do everything I could possibly do. I wanted to have fun with my friends, so I drank too much and didn't pay close enough attention to what I was eating and how much medication I was taking. Times like these can often result in low blood sugar if I'm not careful. One of the things I've had to learn the hard way over the years is that any time I travel or move, any time I'm in a situation that adds stress or anxiety to my life or changes my regular schedule, I need to make a point of being especially diligent about my habits and aware of how my body is reacting.

I remember some of my friends coming to see me in the hospital, and I was more upset about the fact that they weren't out enjoying themselves than I was about myself. I was in excellent hands at the hospital. In fact, it was one of the best-run hospitals I've ever seen, and I've seen a few. When someone needed something, the nurses would literally run to their bedside—not just walk quickly but run. Eventually I was fine that time too, but I was sick enough that David, who happened to be in China already on a business trip, came to get me so we could travel home together. It wasn't the birthday trip I'd envisioned, but that didn't stop me from wanting to travel more in the future. I believe there's always some new experience out there waiting for me, and I'm determined to collect as many of them as I can.

For our twenty-fifth wedding anniversary, David had the number "25" printed in the middle of a big piece of poster board, and then around it he listed all the incredible things we'd done together during those years. He had it framed and gave it to me as a present.

Among the things he listed was the time we rang the bell together at the New York Stock Exchange in 1997, when Yum! Brands (then called Tricon) was founded. And then we did it again in 2012 when he was named CEO of the Year by *Chief Executive* magazine. Not many couples get to do that once let alone twice in their lifetimes.

Back when I was a regular tennis player, I got to hit balls with the legendary Billie Jean King when she came to stay with us at our house in Wichita. We went to probably fifteen Final Four games together, including when the University of Louisville won the National Championship. We got to see the Dallas Cowboys win the Super Bowl when we lived in Dallas, and we saw the Pittsburgh Steelers win a Super Bowl when we lived in Pittsburgh.

We'd seen just about every major Broadway musical that had been staged during those twenty-five years. We went to the Oscars one year because Pepsi was a sponsor, and we even brought

Ashley along. David listed many of the places we'd traveled to, the parties that we'd thrown together, the special occasions that we'd marked as a family.

It's one of the best presents that I've ever received because it's a testament to how rich and full our lives have been. Diabetes or no diabetes, we've had the kind of lives that anyone would feel blessed to have.

Chapter 7

PERSEVERANCE

SOMETIMES I FEEL LIKE A CAT who has been granted nine lives—at least nine, maybe even more. I've certainly had my share of difficult times and experienced some real tests of my endurance. My pregnancy was one. Another came years after when I was on vacation in the Hamptons, of all places.

David and I had gone to visit our friends Barbara and Larry Rafferty at their home in the village of Quogue in the Hamptons. We had spent a wonderful few days together with them and another couple who had also come to stay, Molly and Tim Neher. On our last day in the Hamptons, David left early to go golfing with Larry and Tim, while I stayed behind. The plan was to head to the airport soon after he returned, so in the meantime I busied myself with getting ready to go.

The problems started because my blood sugar was very low that morning. I hadn't yet had the chance to eat anything for breakfast. At the time I was using a new device called a Dexcom glucose monitor, which is a kind of continuous glucose monitor. It didn't require a finger prick test, like I'd always had to do growing up and for many years after, to check the status of my blood sugar. Instead it monitored my glucose levels through a sensor placed just below the skin, which then sent a reading to my phone every few minutes. The ironic thing is that I'd been doing really well on the Dexcom monitor. It had been a game changer for me, helping me remain quite stable most of the time. But that morning, I'd forgotten to charge it. Because of that, and because I was distracted by the fact that we were leaving soon, I didn't realize just how low I'd gotten until I started getting sick to my stomach.

I knew then that I needed to get some orange juice or something to bring my blood sugar back up, but the guest room where we were staying was on the second floor, and there was a steep, narrow set of stairs that I would have to navigate to get to the kitchen. Unsteady as I was, I didn't think I could make it on my own. I don't know why I didn't call for help. Barbara and Molly were both in the house. Asking for help just wasn't something I often did then. In fact, not asking has been the start of many of my problems over the years. Several years before, I had fallen down a flight of stairs at my niece's wedding rehearsal dinner and shattered my ankle because I hadn't asked for assistance. Once, when David and I were skiing in Zurich with his Pepsi colleagues, I didn't want to admit that I couldn't do the last run even though I could barely see a thing and I wasn't a very good skier. I hit an ice patch, went down with a thud, and broke six ribs. I had to fly all the way back to the States in immense pain. Pride and independence are some of my greatest strengths, but sometimes our greatest strengths are also our biggest weaknesses. That was certainly true that day in the Hamptons. Instead of calling for help, I decided to wait for David to get back.

Meanwhile, Barbara and Molly were downstairs wondering what had happened to me. When David returned, they told him I hadn't come down yet. He came straight up to find me and to tell me that he'd moved our departure time up by an hour.

By that time, I'd been sick more than once and was trying my best to get everything cleaned up. David's news that we were leaving early left me a little panicked. While he went back downstairs to tell our hosts what was going on, I started rushing to get ready. I had just pulled the sheets off the bed and still had my arms full of them when I caught my foot on an Oriental rug and went flying into the wall—headfirst.

As I hit the wall, I heard something crack. I knew it wasn't good, but I really didn't have a clue how bad the injury was at that point. In fact, after I called to David and he came back into the room, I told him not to let my neck lock up, so he was massaging my shoulders and moving my head around for me. Unbeknownst to both of us, that was probably the last thing we should have been doing.

Somehow we managed to pull ourselves together, and I made it down the stairs, leaning on David's arm for help, where our friends were waiting for us. They were concerned about me, but we decided it was best just to get home, so David and I said our goodbyes and headed to the airport. It was on the flight that the pain really got to me. I have a high tolerance for pain, but still, it was debilitatingly bad. By the time we landed in Louisville, the flight crew had already radioed ahead. I was carried off the plane on a stretcher, and we went straight to the hospital.

The first reaction from the doctor at the hospital was that he couldn't believe I'd flown home after the injury I'd sustained. Then, in the coming days, I had no fewer than six doctors tell me how lucky I was that it hadn't been worse. "I'm not sure I feel so lucky right now," I told them after I learned that I had a broken neck, but they explained to me that I'd broken my C1 vertebrae, which sits at the top of the neck just beneath the skull, right next to brain matter, which could have left me paralyzed or worse. The fact that I wasn't paralyzed made me seem "lucky" in their eyes, but I couldn't help but think that what would have been really lucky is if none of this had happened in the first place!

I also think that when they said that about my injury, they weren't thinking about just how long and how complicated my recovery would turn out to be. It seemed like one thing after another went wrong after that.

THE HALLUCINATIONS ARE WHAT I remember the most about that time. In fact, many of them are still so vivid in my mind, which is crazy when you consider that none of it actually happened. I remember waking up in the hospital and having no idea where I was, which in and of itself was pretty scary, but then my brain started making up terrifying stories about what was happening around me. At one point I thought that David had put me up in a bed-and-breakfast. I also thought that he was running a drug cartel out of this bed-and-breakfast and that he would invite people to shows he was holding every night, where an audience member would drop through a trap door into the basement and then be killed. I was certain I could hear it happening each time through the walls. I even started calling David "the raven" because he would wear this black hoodie when it got cold in the room, and to my eyes, it made him look like a sinister figure.

One time David walked into my room and gave me a kiss, and I had to ask him who he was because I didn't have a clue. Ashley remembers me talking to her about some sort of creature that I could see sitting on her shoulder. It must have been difficult for them, and it was completely disorienting for me. The hospital staff kept having to move me to different rooms because I would yell that I didn't feel safe. They even had to put me on a feeding tube at one point because I refused to eat after becoming convinced that someone was trying to poison me. I was certain that everyone in the hospital was trying to kill me, and more than anything I wanted to get out of that place. One night I even pulled the IVs out of my arm and tried to escape. I remember someone, probably a nurse or an orderly, remarking, "Wow, she's strong for her size," as they restrained me. When I woke up later, there were two guards stationed outside my door to make sure I didn't try it again.

No one knew what was happening at first. Luckily there was a doctor there who was convinced the hallucinations and disorientation were caused by one of the medications I was on, gabapentin, which I was taking for pain. He said it was a matter of finding the right cocktail of drugs that would work for me, but first they had to wean me off what I was taking. That process took longer than usual because my kidneys weren't able to process the medication as efficiently as they might have if it weren't for my diabetes. All in all, it took about three weeks to come out of my confused and paranoid state. It was awful feeling so completely out of control, and if there is a lesson that I learned from the experience, it's that I never, ever want to feel like that again.

One of the worst parts of it all was not being able to participate in my own care and recovery for so long. There was a doctor at the hospital who wanted to put me in a halo right after it happened, which is a kind of brace used to stabilize the neck. But it's an extreme option that requires drilling into your skull. Because it's anchored that way, you can't just take it off when you need a break. It would have severely limited my mobility, and I can only imagine how uncomfortable it would have been.

Thankfully, I had (and still have) two very powerful people in my corner: my husband and my daughter. One day when David walked into my hospital room, they were already measuring me for the halo. I was terrified because I didn't understand what they were doing. David was not happy about what was happening, so he found the doctor and asked him how he would like it if someone put a device like that on his wife without talking to him first. He thought that being stuck in the halo would break my spirit, and I think he was right. Thankfully, David met with another neurosurgeon to talk about less extreme solutions, and they decided to try a removable neck brace. It worked just fine.

Everyone needs advocates who will be on their side when they're dealing with health issues. I am extremely lucky to have such good ones on my side willing to navigate through complex situations and speak up for me when I can't do it myself.

After my medications had been sorted out and my neck was stabilized, I was sent home, only to return again soon after because I suffered a stroke.

The doctors explained that where I broke my neck, at the base of the skull, there are two arteries that supply blood to the brain. One of those arteries was damaged when I fell, which caused a dissection to form, which basically means it tore and began to bleed. When bleeding happens, the body naturally forms blood clots, and when a blood clot broke off and traveled to my brain, it impeded the flow of blood. That's when the stroke happened.

What made me really feel lucky was the fact that David and Ashley even caught it at all. With a stroke, the sooner you dis-cover it the better, but because my neck was going to take months to heal, I was on a lot of pain medication and spending most of my time in bed sleeping. I already wasn't acting like my usual self, so it would be hard for anyone to pick up on the telltale signs. When they saw my face start to droop on one side, however, they knew something was very wrong and rushed me back to the hospital.

After that, I couldn't talk very well for a while, and it was just another thing I had to recover from after everything I'd been through already.

Symptoms of a Stroke

My daughter, Ashley, always said after that episode that she wished she'd been better informed about what to look for to determine if someone is having a stroke, especially since time is of the essence when it happens. The CDC recommends that people administer the Act F.A.S.T. test if they suspect someone might be having a stroke, which has four basic parts:

F—Face: Ask the person to smile. Does one side of the face droop?

A—Arms: Ask the person to raise both arms. Does one arm drift downward?

S—Speech: Ask the person to repeat a simple phrase. Is the speech slurred or strange?

T—Time: If you see any of these signs, call 911 right away.

ALL TOLD, I SPENT ABOUT TWO AND A HALF months in the hospital that summer. There was so much going on that I didn't even realize until the end of that period that I had also broken thirteen teeth when I ran into the wall. Because there had been more pressing concerns to deal with, no one had paid much attention to them. When I started to feel like myself again, I looked in the mirror and was shocked and angry to discover the sorry state of my teeth! By that point, most of them were beyond saving. After I got through everything else, I had to have eleven implants to fix them, and it was a while before I could eat solid foods again. It took at least four months for my broken neck to really start to heal. I had to wear a neck brace all that time. Then there were the lingering effects of the stroke. One side was weaker than the other, as happens with strokes, and I would drag my foot a little on that side. It could be difficult to walk, and my balance was affected. Many of the lingering effects were small things, but they drove me crazy. My recovery was complicated by my waning eyesight, which could also make me unsteady on my feet, and the last thing I needed was to fall again. Through it all, though, I was determined to come back from the experience, and I worked hard in physical therapy to make it happen. I'm proud to say that I fought through it and, in time, got my functioning back.

It was a long road back, and part of the challenge was due to the unique nature of my injury but some of it was due to the effects of diabetes. Wounds tend to heal more slowly when you have diabetes. Medications can affect you differently. Then there's the fact that you have to continue to manage your diabetes in tandem with whatever other treatments and care you're receiving.

As is true for so many health conditions, none of this gets easier as you age. You may have noticed me writing more and more about low blood sugar episodes. My endocrinologist once explained that, as I got older, my brain got more and more used to the experience of having low blood sugar. As a result, I wouldn't always feel the symptoms until my levels dropped to such a low level that I was already in the danger zone and maybe even passed out. At that point, it's obviously too late to respond on my own. The phenomenon even has a name: hypoglycemia unawareness. It basically means that your internal warning system starts to falter and you're less able to tell when your blood sugar is running low.

I've had to make tough choices over the years for the sake of my health, and it hasn't always been easy. My eyesight diminished after I gave birth to Ashley, but I got enough of it back after all the eye surgeries that I was able to function just like I had before. For a while, at least. I was able to drive again, for example, and continued to do so all through Ashley's childhood and well past the time she left home. However, my sight continued to decline slowly but steadily over the years. When I was in my late fifties, I had two near-accidents, both of them close calls. By then I could hardly see at all out of my right eye, which was the more damaged of the two, and I walked away from those experiences feeling shook up. No one forced me to do it, but I felt like I had to make the call to give up my driver's license.

I cried when I finally did it. I knew what I was giving up. Being able to drive is a symbol of freedom and independence, and that wasn't an easy thing to let go of. So I let myself cry for a bit, and then I asked myself what I was going to do to make things better for myself. I started by making a list of friends who would be willing to take me places and car services I could call when I needed to go somewhere. One summer, when we were staying in the Hamptons, I decided I was going to get to know the area by visiting all the local farmer's markets. To do that, I called up several girlfriends and made a date with a different one each week to visit a new market. It was a way to continue living life the way I wanted to despite what I'd had to give up. And I got a chance to have a lot of fun with some great people in the process.

I'm not saying it's always easy. Some days I still wish I could just get in my car, drive myself to the grocery store, and buy myself a donut to eat right then and there. It can be tough to let go of things, not because you want to but because you know it's better for you, and it can feel like a real test of your resilience when you do. What I've come to learn, however, is that flexibility and resilience go hand in hand. Diabetes may have its rules that need to be followed, but if you're willing to bend and adapt, there are always ways to continue to experience the joys in life, no matter what life throws at you.

Hypoglycemia Unawareness

Repeated episodes of low blood sugar can, over time, result in hypoglycemia unawareness, which is when a person can no longer pick up on the early warning signs like heart palpitation, shakiness, dizziness, sweating, or fatigue. It's important to talk to your doctor if this happens as it may require changes to your treatment.

Chapter 8

RENEWAL

I'VE LIVED WITH DIABETES for more than sixty years now. During that time, so much has changed about the way the condition is understood and treated. I've gone from using insulin derived from animals to using synthetic insulin that comes in a wide variety of forms, from rapid acting to long lasting, that doctors can choose from to best suit the unique needs of their patients.

I've gone from periodically peeing on paper test strips to test my blood sugar to having a glucose monitor that attaches to my skin and tracks it for me, sending the info straight to my smartphone on a regular basis.

I've gone from using old-fashioned steel needles to give myself shots on a set schedule to using an insulin pump in what's called a "closed-loop system" that combines a continuous glucose monitor with a pump that automatically delivers insulin as needed. People sometimes call this system an artificial pancreas because it aims to mimic the work the pancreas would do if it functioned normally.

It's amazing to think that kind of technology is possible today given that diabetes was considered a death sentence not so very long ago. It's also amazing to think how lucky I've been on my journey with diabetes. My dad was among the first people to receive insulin treatment for his condition, which meant he was able to live a relatively normal life, holding down a good job and having a wife and family, things that would have been impossible a generation before him. Because I grew up in a family that had some understanding of the condition, I was lucky enough to be diagnosed right away when I developed diabetes and to receive treatment for it. And then, as I've gotten older, I've been lucky enough to be in position where I can take advantage of all the new developments that have made treating diabetes easier and more consistent even while, far too often, the lifesaving drugs and technologies that people with diabetes need are too expensive and inaccessible for too many people.

It's a gift to be able to look back on my life and feel this lucky. I'm a big believer in the idea that if you look for the lessons in life, you will always find something you can learn from, something that will help you grow, and something that can have a positive impact on your life. Because of that, I see diabetes as not only one of the biggest challenges I've faced in my life but also a source of some of my greatest gifts.

There can even be silver linings in living with diabetes, as there often are when we face challenges in our lives. It's hard for me to imagine what my life would have been like if I hadn't had this condition, but I do know that it has taught me a few things over the years, like how to be strong, adaptable, and resilient. I think it has helped me develop empathy for people in difficult circumstances.

It may sound odd to some, but even after all these years, I'm still finding silver linings.

Not so long ago, I was having trouble maintaining my balance. My doctor told me I had spinal stenosis at the site where I had broken my neck years earlier. He recommended spinal surgery to stabilize the area, help with my balance, and relieve some of the pain. I was nervous about having surgery on my spine, but I made the decision to do it anyway. The surgery went well, I made it through recovery, and I was diligently doing all my physical therapy to fight my way back when a major setback happened.

It was in February of 2020, just as the world was shutting down from Covid-19, that I had a severe hypoglycemic seizure while at home with David. I'd been having a lot of neck pain that day, so I took a sleeping pill. That was after drinking my usual two glasses of wine. It's strange that, in all my years of living with diabetes, I'd never heard the warnings about sleeping pills, but unfortunately, I hadn't. I know now that sleeping aids can be dangerous for people with diabetes because if the person experiences a low, or what's called nocturnal or nighttime hypoglycemia, they're less likely to be woken up by symptoms telling them they need to take action quickly.

The ideal blood glucose range can be different for different people, but I always knew that if my blood sugar fell below 50 mg/dL, I would feel lightheaded and not totally cognizant of what was happening around me. (For many people, that happens when their levels fall below 70 mg/dL.) On that night, my blood sugar went as low as 20 mg/dL, which is crisis territory.

I started having a seizure while I slept, but I didn't wake up. It just so happened that our dog, Sarge, was having medical issues of his own that night, so David stayed downstairs with him and wasn't nearby to pick up on what was happening to me. That meant I experienced a seizure and dangerously low blood sugar for at least five hours before he came upstairs in the morning and found me.

He called an ambulance right away, and I spent ten days in the hospital after that. I don't remember any of it. Not him finding me. Not the time I spent in the hospital. Apparently, there were questions about whether my cognition would come back or if I had permanent damage, but I don't remember those discussions either. I don't remember a single thing until after I came home from the hospital.

I had been on an insulin pump prior to the seizure, but after I returned from the hospital, my doctor advised that I should avoid getting back on it right away. My brain was still healing from what had happened, so the doctor didn't think it was a good idea for me to have that degree of control over my insulin. If I wasn't in a totally lucid state, I could accidentally give myself the wrong amount, which could have serious consequences. So instead, we went back to basics. The doctor set up an injection schedule, just like I'd had when I was younger, and David had to learn on the fly how to manage my treatment for me. He kept me on track and administered all my shots.

The situation was made even more complicated by the fact that these were the early days of Covid. Tents were being set up in the hospital parking lot to create a testing center at the same time that I was inside in the ICU. When I was discharged from the hospital, David and Ashley had to consider whether to bring in nurses to help with my care given the current circumstances. Because diabetes is one of the conditions that makes contracting Covid even more dangerous, my doctor advised against it. Having people coming in and out of the house would only increase our exposure, so it was recommended that we quarantine as best we could. That meant that it fell almost entirely to David to make sure I was getting what I needed until I was well enough to take care of myself again.

Being cared for by my husband in that way was a new experience for me. I'd never let him be part of managing my condition before. I had never even wanted him to know too much about it or ask me too many questions. I always thought of diabetes as my disease, and I never wanted anyone controlling my care but me. One of the first things I remember saying to him after I started to return to my old self again, was: "You're giving me shots? How did that happen!?" He explained to me that I hadn't been able to take care of myself, so he had to step up. He didn't have a choice.

I wasn't as upset about it as I would have expected. Even though I'd always been adamant about managing things myself,

I found I was happy to learn that he knew how to do it too. After managing on my own for so long, it suddenly felt like something we could share. And he did such a good job that it made me fall in love with him all over again.

I know it was a really hard time for him. It wasn't a simple recovery. Later, I had another stroke. And then another seizure. I had to fight through more issues with my medications. For a while there, David thought he had lost me, and it wasn't the last time he would think that. There was so much that he had to handle on his own during such a scary time. I can tell by the look he gets in his eyes when he talks about it that it really was difficult. I feel so sorry for that. And yet, once again, we found one of those unexpected silver linings: in the end, we both believe that time brought us closer together.

That wasn't the only thing I gained from that experience either. Sometimes our most difficult moments can be the impetus for real change. After all, it can be difficult to make changes in our lives when everything's comfortable and going well. It's the moments of pain or fear or loss that so often drive us to examine ourselves and motivate us to do things differently.

That's what happened to me after my seizure. It's scary to feel like you have lost your cognitive ability. It's incredible to think that I was completely unaware that Covid was even happening until David explained it to me weeks later. To have so much going on all around me and to not understand or remember any of it is very unsettling.

When I first started coming back to cognition, I didn't know what had happened exactly, but I did have this persistent feeling like I had done something terrible. I didn't remember the sleeping pill I had taken or the wine I had drunk, but I had this sense that I'd caused my seizure myself. I felt horrible guilt about it, especially because of how it affected my family. That feeling stuck around for months, and I couldn't escape it.

The shock of it all propelled me to do something pretty drastic: I gave up alcohol once and for all. At least two glasses of wine a night was typical for me before all this happened. I would pour one for dinner and then have another afterward. I'd been a regular drinker since college, which means it was a habit that I'd maintained for decades by then. I think I always figured that since it was a ritual that was good enough for my dad, who had a drink every night as soon as he got home from work, it was good enough for me too. Except for the months when I was pregnant, I drank every night, just like my dad did, for more than forty years.

It was the idea that I could permanently lose my cognitive ability that really did it for me. The very idea scared me enough that I never wanted to drink again.

The funny thing is that, after doing things the same way for so long, I don't even miss it now. I've found that I love being sober. I've never felt better. I'm more clearheaded. I have a more positive outlook. I feel more present in my life. I've even come around to feeling grateful for the experience I went through that inspired me to make this change. Because without it, I'd probably still be having my two drinks a night, and I'd have never known what life could be like without them.

I feel freer now too. It wasn't like I got drunk on a regular basis, but I had come to rely on my evening ritual. I would sometimes play these games with myself, saying that I wasn't reliant on alcohol because I never drank before five o'clock at night. But come five o'clock, I always had my drink without fail. That was my pattern. That was my dad's pattern. That's quite a pattern to break, but I had this earth-shattering motive, so I was able to do it. I guess it's never too late to make changes in your life, especially when they're changes for the better.

EVEN THOUGH DAVID GOT REALLY GOOD at monitoring my blood sugar and giving me my shots, there came a time as I continued to heal when I wanted to get back on the insulin pump. I wanted to do it not only because it gave me more independence but also because, when you know how to work it properly, it provides more consistency and stability. Of course, like with all new technologies, there's a learning curve. I had to relearn how to work it, and in the process, I made a few mistakes.

The first night I was back on it, I gave myself about twenty units of insulin, which is way too much. I accidentally pushed the wrong button, and there was no going back after that. The only thing I could do was start eating to compensate for the extra insulin. I downed six Cokes in a row and ate a bunch of stuff. My stomach didn't feel so great afterward, but I managed to level off without having to go to the hospital.

After that David wanted me to get rid of the pump and go back to the old way of giving myself shots. He was afraid that I was going to make another mistake, one that might kill me next time. But I insisted that we could do this and that the pump was the right choice. Now neither one of us can imagine being without it because my blood sugar readings are nearly perfect almost all the time, probably better than they've ever been in my life.

That's what's working for me today, but if my condition changes or if the technology continues to improve, I know I'll adapt. I know from experience that I can learn new things and get back up after I've been knocked down. It can be humbling to have diabetes. It can feel overwhelming at times. Sometimes it can seem like so much is out of your control and that simple mistakes can have big consequences. But it's important to remember, I think, that life can feel like that for everyone at times. Everyone has their challenges. Diabetes has been a lifelong one for me, but that has never stopped me from having what I consider to be an amazing life.

Sixty-plus years I've lived with diabetes, and I wouldn't trade my life for anyone's.

GIVING BACK

MY DAD ALWAYS TOLD ME that I could do anything anyone else could do as long as I followed the rules of diabetes. It was a powerful message, one that I took to heart over the course of my life. I grew up believing that I could have any life I wanted and that diabetes did not need to stand in my way.

At the same time, those rules that were imposed on me because of this condition are things that I've really struggled with at times. I still have vivid memories of the food battles my mom and I had when I was growing up. I remember the feeling of wanting to break free from what was always, always, relentlessly expected of me by sneaking candy on my way home from school, for example, or running a little wild when I got to college. These may seem like pretty normal types of rebellion that kids go through as they assert their independence, but for me they carried additional weight, an extra element of risk, because of my diabetes.

It has been tricky to navigate that line between following the rules and not allowing those rules to feel like limits on my potential to live a life of my own making. It's something I've worked at throughout my entire life, and I admit that I haven't always gotten the balance right. I used to feel bad about that. I felt bad when I did something that in my mind made me a "bad diabetic." I kept secrets about those behaviors so that no one would judge me. But at some point in my life, I had to admit to myself that none of us is perfect, nor can we be expected to be. And if there are no perfect people, then there's certainly no such thing as a "perfect diabetic."

At the end of the day, I think my struggles with diabetes can be taken as a metaphor for life in general because the cycle is the same no matter what we do: We try our best. We make mistakes. We pick ourselves back up when we fall. And then we try again. And again. And again. The best thing any of us can do is to allow that cycle to happen without beating ourselves up when we falter. After all, we have enough to deal with without feeling bad about our inevitable imperfections.

It's with these ideas in the back of my mind that I've been thinking lately about my dad's sentiment, which defined how I thought about my diabetes while I was growing up and long into adulthood. We're all unique people, and we all need to find our own way on this journey. But to help others as much as I can, I put together my own list of "rules" for living with diabetes. I use quotation marks around the word "rules" because I was never the best at following rules and because everyone's experience is going to be different. In fact, I think a better word would be something like "guidelines" or "tips" to indicate that these are things to aim for rather than hard-and-fast rules that can never be broken. They also have more to do with how you see yourself and the meaning you place on having this condition than with any medical aspects. That's because first, I'm not a doctor, and any specific medical advice should only come from experts on this condition; and second, I believe that what it means to you to have diabetes is as important has how you manage it.

With that in mind, here are some of the top tips that have worked for me—most of the time, at least. I hope they can serve as guideposts as you figure out how you, too, can live a full and happy life while navigating the realities, challenges, and possibilities of having diabetes.

Wendy's Tips for Living with Diabetes

1. Recognize that diabetes is not the end of your life.

2. Learn how to be self-reliant and take responsibility for your condition.

3. Stay as active as possible because a strong body can help you weather setbacks.

4. Don't beat yourself up over your mistakes—learn from them and move forward.

5. Remember to give yourself credit for facing the challenges that come with this condition and know that they make you stronger and more resilient.

6. Embrace life like everyone else, knowing that it is full of possibilities.

7. Be proud but don't let your pride get in your way. My pride has been a stumbling block and has led to some of my biggest mistakes.

8. Don't be afraid to ask for help when you need it.

9. Help your family get educated about how to support you and handle potential crisis situations.

10. Set up a partnership with medical professionals because managing diabetes is a team effort.

11. Adapt to new technologies. It's worth the effort because new advancements are making life easier and easier for people with diabetes.

12. Stay optimistic because you never know what's right around the corner!

It truly is a gift to be able to look back on my life and feel this lucky. It's partly because we've been so blessed that my family decided to do something to help people like me. I know from experience that the lifesaving and life-affirming care that people with diabetes need is often far too expensive and difficult to come by for too many people. The Wendy Novak Diabetes Institute (formerly the Wendy Novak Diabetes Center), which is part of Norton Children's Endocrinology and affiliated with the University of Louisville School of Medicine, started as a Christmas present. My husband, David, and my daughter, Ashley, figured they could give me no bigger and better gift than helping to fund a place where children and young adults in our community can get the help they need to live long, healthy, and active lives with diabetes.

I suppose you could even say that diabetes has given my whole family a sense of purpose, which is how our support for the institute came about. Ashley, who now does nonprofit work as the executive director of our Lift a Life Novak Family Foundation, remembers feeling like she wanted to do something to help people with diabetes ever since the seventh grade when she had to call an ambulance because I was suffering from a low blood sugar episode. Our partnership with Norton Healthcare has enabled us to do just that.

I have always been certain about the value of this endeavor, but in the beginning I wasn't so sure about the name. Initially, it just didn't feel like me to have "Wendy Novak" written in big letters across a building somewhere. But I've found that even this has led to unexpected gifts.

Not long ago, I was having my hair cut when my longtime hairdresser mentioned that she knew a little boy who wanted to meet me. His name is Alexander Berres, and he knows who I am because he has diabetes, too, and receives care at the institute bearing my name.

It was a happy accident that my hairdresser was able to put us in touch. I called Alexander on his tenth birthday, sang him "Happy Birthday," and talked with him about how I was diagnosed with diabetes when I was about his age. It was such a joy to hear about how much he loved the atmosphere at the institute and how good he felt about the care he was receiving there. It wasn't a long conversation, but he called it the biggest thrill of his life. I have to admit, it was a thrill for me, too, to be able to have that kind of impact on someone.

Through the institute, I've had a chance to meet with families of newly diagnosed kids, who sometimes think that what's happening to them is a real tragedy. I understand their feelings and how frightening it can be when something like this happens, especially to your children, but I hope that people also come to understand that it really isn't the end of the world. Children with diabetes can live full, happy, productive lives. I hope my life story, as told in these pages, can stand as proof of that fact.

My own mother once said, "I don't know if having to deal with diabetes makes you a special person or not, but the two people in my life with diabetes, my husband and my daughter, have both been such special people. For them to have it has not been the worst experience, and I feel so lucky to have had them in my life." I hope all children with this condition and their family members can come to think of it in this way.

ACKNOWLEDGMENTS

FIRST AND FOREMOST want to express my immense gratitude to my father, Jack Henderson. He prayed to God that I would never have diabetes. Yet he helped me through it, and I watched him live his life to the fullest. Diabetes never defined my dad, and it doesn't define me. He gave me the gift of that mindset.

I also wish to thank my mother, Ann Henderson, for her love and support. You managed a large family and had a chronically ill child, yet you never set limitations on what I could achieve. When I think about how the Wendy Novak Diabetes Institute can support families, I think of you and how you had to learn on your own without the support of a medical team. Thank you for learning.

I also want to thank my siblings. I know I often got the candy, and you didn't, but thank you for still loving me. Cindy, I love your family-oriented heart. Jeff, you are honest, hardworking, and kind. Rick, you take great care of your family. Gretchen, you are giving and loving to everyone around you. As we grow older, I am thankful for your friendship and support.

I also want to thank Jean and Charles Novak. You welcomed me into your family like I was your own. You could have put a damper on my romance with David, but you knew our love was true. I am forever grateful.

Thank you to Christa Bourg for your literary mastery of my story and your inquisitive way of mining my nuggets of wisdom to give hope to others with diabetes. I am thankful for your writing gift and your friendship. Thank you to Alli and Janet at Disruption Books for your guidance and care with my story. Thank you to Janet Lambert for your care and support. Thank you to Dr. Kupper Wintergerst and the entire Wendy Novak Diabetes Institute for coming into my life and presenting a vision for changing the experience of diabetes care in our hometown and nation. We believe in you and the vision you have for a future without diabetes. Let's continue to move to No. 1 in the nation.

Finally, I want to thank my small but mighty family.

My husband, David, for falling hard for me and loving me with that same intensity for the last forty-eight years. This book was a labor of love for both of us, and your encouragement and support during the writing journey meant so much to me. Our hours of reading chapters and rewriting the story is something I will cherish forever. You were right, I do have a story to tell, and you helped me to share it in such a meaningful way. I love you and you know . . .

My dear Ashley "Sweetie" Brooke, thank you for helping me to publish my story. I dedicated your life to God when you were born, and I have enjoyed watching you shine as you grow into an adult and a mother of your own beautiful children. You were worth every part of my journey, and I love you. Jonathan, thank you for loving Ashley well. I am glad I said yes. My lovely grandchildren, Audrey, Claire, and Luke, you are delightfully fun to live with and love. I enjoy every second we are together.

ABOUT THE
INSTITUTE

THE GOAL OF THE Wendy Novak Diabetes Institute is to become a national center of excellence by expanding and elevating diabetes care services across the region while helping children and adults with diabetes manage their conditions. The institute will support continued coordination between care teams to ensure seamless continuity for pediatric patients as they grow and move on to adult care.

In 2013, an initial gift of $5 million to the Norton Healthcare Foundation established the Wendy Novak Diabetes Center, which focused on pediatric care. The Lift a Life Novak Family Foundation built on this in 2022 with a $15 million gift that transformed the center into the Wendy Novak Diabetes Institute, which continues to offer treatment and education to thousands of young adults and expands the scope of care to patients from childhood to adulthood. This gift is the starting point of a

$60 million vision to expand diabetes care for children and adults as well as build the top diabetes institute in the country.

Pediatric care at the Wendy Novak Diabetes Institute is a service of Norton Healthcare, which is recognized as having one of the nation's top diabetes programs. The hospital is listed sixteenth in *U.S. News & World Report*'s 2022 rankings for organizations specializing in pediatric diabetes and endocrinology. The program ranked eighteenth in 2020 and 2021, fueled by funding from the Lift a Life Novak Family Foundation.

Pediatric outpatient services for the Wendy Novak Diabetes Institute are housed in the Novak Center for Children's Health, a 176,000-square-foot outpatient medical center in downtown Louisville, Kentucky, that gives children and families easy access to Norton Healthcare Endocrinology, which is affiliated with the University of Louisville School of Medicine, as well as additional pediatric specialists and primary care providers. Located two blocks from Norton Healthcare, the Novak Center for Children's Health is one of the largest and most technically advanced pediatric outpatient centers in the country, with over thirty specialists housed in one location. Pediatric inpatient care is provided at Jack & Wendy's Place, located within Norton Healthcare.

Adult outpatient services are offered through the Norton Community Medical Associates endocrinology offices, while inpatient services are provided at Norton Healthcare hospitals.

MAKE A DIFFERENCE

To find out how you can help, visit wendynovakdiabetesinstitute.com/make-a-difference.

ABOUT THE AUTHOR

WENDY LOUISE NOVAK has lived with type 1 diabetes since she was seven years old. It's a condition that runs in her family, and when her father, Jack Henderson, was diagnosed at the age of four, it was considered by many to be a death sentence. Despite those dire predictions, Jack lived to be seventy-two. Thanks to advances in medical treatments and a resilient spirit, Wendy, too, has lived with diabetes for more than sixty years—and more than just lived with it, she has thrived.

Because it has always been important to Wendy that everyone has a chance to reach their full potential, no matter what obstacles stand in their way, in 1999, she and her husband, David Novak, established the Lift a Life Novak Family Foundation, which provides grants in the areas of leadership development, hunger relief, early childhood education, and military family support. In 2022, the foundation helped establish the Wendy Novak Diabetes Institute, a service of Norton Healthcare, in Louisville, Kentucky, in order to expand and elevate diabetes care throughout the region for children and adults.

Wendy currently serves as an advisory board member for the Wendy Novak Diabetes Institute and chair of her family foundation's Community Impact Grant Committee. She also serves on the board of Camp Hendon, a camp for children with diabetes that she was lucky enough to attend as a child.

Wendy holds a bachelor's degree in journalism from the University of Missouri and a master's degree in social work from Columbia University. Last but far from least, she is the proud mother of Ashley and grandmother of Audrey, Claire, and Luke.